Emerging Infectious Diseases
Art in Science

POLYXENI POTTER

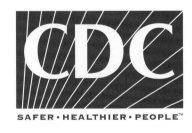

SAFER · HEALTHIER · PEOPLE™

CENTERS FOR DISEASE
CONTROL AND PREVENTION

OXFORD
UNIVERSITY PRESS

Oxford University Press is a department of the University of Oxford.
It furthers the University's objective of excellence in research,
scholarship, and education by publishing worldwide.

Oxford   New York
Auckland   Cape Town   Dar es Salaam   Hong Kong   Karachi
Kuala Lumpur   Madrid   Melbourne   Mexico City   Nairobi
New Delhi   Shanghai   Taipei   Toronto

With offices in
Argentina   Austria   Brazil   Chile   Czech Republic   France   Greece
Guatemala   Hungary   Italy   Japan   Poland   Portugal   Singapore
South Korea   Switzerland   Thailand   Turkey   Ukraine   Vietnam

Oxford is a registered trade mark of Oxford University Press
in the UK and certain other countries.

Published in the United States of America by
Oxford University Press
198 Madison Avenue, New York, NY 10016

Catalog record is available from the Library of Congress.
ISBN 978-0-19-931569-7

9 8 7 6 5 4 3 2
Printed in China by
Asia Pacific Offset

Oxford University Press is proud to pay a portion of its sales for this book to the CDC Foundation. Chartered by Congress, the CDC
Foundation began operations in 1995 as an independent, nonprofit organization fostering support for CDC through public-private
partnerships. Further information about the CDC Foundation can be found at www.cdcfoundation.org. The CDC Foundation did not
prepare any portion of this book and is not responsible for its contents.

Contents

Foreword

Does the world need yet another art book? In a word, yes. In fact, it desperately needs a great many more art books. As Yogi Berra pointed out, it is déjà vu all over again.

When the infectious disease leadership at the Centers for Disease Control and Prevention posed a similar question in the early 1990s, they wondered whether the world needed yet another infectious disease journal. They had some help in addressing the question. That help came to them in the landmark 1992 Institute of Medicine report, *Emerging Infections—Microbial Threats to Health in the United States*, edited by Nobel Laureate Joshua Lederberg, arbovirologist Robert Shope, and microbiologist Stanley C. Oaks Jr. Although other infectious disease and microbiology journals existed and flourished, none filled the public health niche that was desperately vacant in the era when untreatable AIDS was raging, tuberculosis was reemerging, and antimicrobial drug-resistant organisms were gaining a foothold in the health care and community setting.

By taking as its mission to inform the academic and public health communities about emerging infections, the fledgling *Emerging Infectious Diseases* journal adopted a broad scope, one that encompassed not only clinical medicine and epidemiology but also microbiology, veterinary medicine, social science, and even the humanities. Taking the view that readers were public health oriented meant that they needed actionable information that they otherwise had little time to access or even read.

Although infectious disease may arguably be called the most successful medical specialty in history, microbes continually evolve and adapt to novel hosts, new geographic places, or climatic conditions. That is the challenge *Emerging Infectious Diseases* readers face; emergence is a never-ending process when it applies to infectious diseases. As Dr. Lederberg was fond of saying, "It's their genes versus our wits."

The contents of *Emerging Infectious Diseases* cover the global waterfront. Nearly every issue has reports from nations on nearly all the continents, and articles address human and animal infections related to all major categories of organisms. The news is often not good, and analyses of the morbidity and mortality paint a bleak picture. Since its earliest years, the journal's editors sought to communicate more than the epidemiologic and pathologic findings. They, largely led by Managing Editor Poly Potter, wanted to depict the human aspect of emerging infections—from pain and death to nobility and triumph. What better way to do this than to place the human aspect right up front? The first few years of the journal's publishing history reflect a certain amount of experimentation—the initial covers merely listing the table of contents and cautiously moving toward color images, and more recent issues representing the concept in full bloom. A cross section of covers and accompanying essays are included in this book.

As with its scientific scope, *Emerging Infectious Diseases* adopted a broad view of art, seeking out images from artists from all nations, eras of history (from prehistoric to contemporary), genres, and schools of art, and as many media as the two-dimensional print covers can accommodate.

Poly Potter has done a great service to the emerging infections community of scientists. By assembling a collection of covers and essays, she has been more than responsive to a frequent query: "Why don't you publish a book of those beautiful covers?" The question is now answered, and the goal of the book is less to review the past than it is to stimulate thought about the future. We thought that the world really did need one more art book, and we are glad that you found this one.

D. Peter Drotman
Editor-in-Chief
Emerging Infectious Diseases

Preface

ARTS, SCIENCE, AND THE PURSUIT OF KNOWLEDGE

For there will be hard data and they will be hard to understand
For the trivial will trap you and the important escape you
For the Committee will be unable to resolve the question
For there will be the arts
   and some will call them
   soft data
   whereas in fact they are the hard data
   by which our lives are lived
     —John Stone, "Gaudeamus Igitur: A Valediction"

John Stone, cardiologist and poet, was an expert on the mechanics of the human heart, inside and out. When he submitted a manuscript for publication in *Emerging Infectious Diseases*, he urged that the cover for that month show a painting by Georges Rouault, *Les Trois Juges* (*The Three Judges*), c. 1936 (page xvii). As the fledgling journal could not afford the copyright fee for this image, he arranged for payment through his own institution, Emory University in Atlanta. The painting, a shock of blood red roughly forming the abstract figures of the judges, made a spectacular splash and a fitting companion to his account of "a man . . . who had walked and worked among us and died of love."

Stone's choice of art for his story about syphilis was unusual. Most authors submitting manuscripts for publication in science journals view art as graphic illustration intended to clarify or summarize, to provide a visual explanation of content: epidemiologic curves, line charts, bar graphs, genomic trees, explicit photographs of lesions, color representations of organisms under the microscope, images of vectors or human and animal anatomic features. Fine art, the creative effort concerned solely with beauty and collected in museums and galleries, is not the authors' usual choice, nor is it often found in science publication.

How did fine art become a cover option for a science journal, and how did Stone know about it? *Emerging Infectious Diseases*, a public health journal published by the Centers for Disease Control and Prevention, has drawn on fine art for its covers nearly since inception in 1995 with the mission to promote the recognition of new and reemerging infections and the understanding of factors involved in their prevention and elimination. Charged with communicating the threat of these diseases, their unpredictable course, and the inevitability of their emergence in time and space, the journal reached out to a global audience from academia, laboratories, clinical practice, public health, social sciences, and other disciplines. Stone was part of this audience.

Intended as a communication tool, not an archive of science, *Emerging Infectious Diseases* was designed to be inclusive rather than exclusive; to demystify public health data: "here is what we found and here is what the findings mean for public health"; and to reach out to a broad audience through electronic communication. These goals called for a reader-friendly format and a unique profile that would enable it to fill a niche left open by well-established, venerable journals in the crowded marketplace. Art was harnessed to elucidate the issues, seek solutions, and engage the general reader in the process of disease prevention and control. As a result, art became irrevocably connected with the journal's unique profile. And, while fine art on the cover of a science journal was not altogether new, linking the art with the science inside was.

In print publishing, the audience can be narrowly defined: public health practitioners in state health departments and academic institutions in the United States and around the world. In electronic publishing, ease of access on the Web expands the audience in unanticipated ways. And whereas print assumes a light spillover of scientific or technical information to the public through the mass media, an electronic product must take into account the expanded audience: patients seeking direct information about illnesses and treatment, students and researchers whose first impulse is to turn to the Web for information, continuing education candidates, and a largely unserved multifaceted international audience.

The diverse composition of its audience influenced both the content and format of *Emerging Infectious Diseases*. A multidisciplinary audience requires definitions explanations, clarifications, substantive editing of submitted articles for readability, and features with broad appeal. "Another Dimension," a section inviting thoughtful essays, short stories, or poems on philosophical issues related to science, medical practice, and human health was created for just this purpose, to explore science and the human condition, fear and pain, the unanticipated side of epidemic investigations, how people perceive and cope with infection and illness. The section is intended to evoke compassion for human suffering and expand the science reader's literary scope. This is the category in which Stone submitted his short story "An Infected Heart."

Images for the cover of *Emerging Infectious Diseases* are selected for artistic quality and communication effectiveness. As the images, drawn from all periods, prehistoric to contemporary, lend their beauty or poignancy to the covers of the journal, they also illustrate ideas, raise consciousness, reveal truth, stimulate the intellect, and fire the emotions. And while they are selected to attract readers, they also surprise, delight, inspire, and enlighten them.

"How are images selected?" For their ability to invoke in the mind of the reader subtle but lasting connections. Connections that unlock understanding, dispel confusion, promote compassion. "According to Brueghel / when Icarus fell / it was spring / a farmer was ploughing / his field / the whole pageantry / of the year was / awake," wrote physician and poet William Carlos Williams in his poem "Landscape with the Fall of Icarus," "unsignificantly / off the coast / there was / a splash quite unnoticed / this was / Icarus drowning." Without imagery, without the brushwork, or the verse, one may never hear the splash of "Icarus drowning," the very point in Brueghel's painting, Williams's poem, and public health research.

"Tell us about it." The cover story, a regular feature used to discuss the artwork and its connection with the contents of the journal, evolved by popular demand, literally out of the readers' wish to *know* the art and how it relates to them and to what they do. The life of the artist, the period, and the work are good for a historical backdrop. Through one of countless possible interpretations, the art moves the discussion toward the human element in the work. The public health topic at hand provides the "hard data," which can always be elucidated in human terms. Suffering is universal. The purpose of scientific endeavor is its alleviation, the betterment of humanity, and the improvement of the quality of life for all people.

The landscape of emerging infections is rife with plagues, from old, familiar ones resurfacing to completely new, unknown ones destined to occupy biomedical research for the rest of time, from malaria resurgence and dengue to SARS, from pandemic flu and poverty-related illness to intentional use of biologic agents and antimicrobial-drug resistance. These plagues cannot be addressed apart from the community, which ultimately funds their investigation just as surely as it provides the surveillance data, the study groups, and the statistical evidence. Public health research can hardly be conceived apart from the human element: the people who become ill.

Art humanizes and enhances science content and educates readers outside their areas of expertise about important unnoticed connections. Art accomplishes this by infusing scientific findings with empathetic understanding—in a literal way, through the faces and places of traditional painting or completely in the abstract through new ways of seeing. Beauty, color, emotion, style, and the eccentricity and vitality associated with the artists' lives and times, against the formality of technical prose, open up the possibility, indeed the capacity, for alternative interpretation of data, by introducing the metaphor. The metaphor, according to Aristotle, owes its strength to making possible "an intuitive perception of the similarity of dissimilars," by implying likeness. A bird is not human, but a single element in its appearance can invoke humanity, just as a single element in a plant's appearance can distinguish its species.

Right and Left (1909), a painting by Winslow Homer (Figure 2), was used on a cover in conjunction with avian influenza. The title is hunt jargon for using a double-barreled gun to shoot two ducks in rapid succession. The hunter, on the waves in some distance, is barely visible behind the flare of the shotgun. The aquatic scene is witnessed from the birds' perspective in the sky. Bird on the right, possibly struck first, falls limply toward the ocean. Bird on the left, in direct range, makes desperate attempt at exit as the second shot is fired. Or is the bird on the left stunned from being hit first, in the back, while the other bird is diving to escape?

The "in your face" travel of the birds and bullets adds dramatic immediacy. Agitated waters, a glaring eye, and the rocking boat underline violence. Dislodged feather and ray of sunshine mark the fleeting moment. This scene, painted near the end of Homer's life when death must have been on his mind, seems the culmination of a lifetime of observation. In a few brushstrokes, the artist delivers the ocean's power, the vastness of creation, conflict in the world, riddles in nature. He projects the birds and their plight, the hunter's unimportance, even as he fires the fatal shots. The ambiguity in their posture is the artist's ambivalence about which bird died first. The threat is imminent and inevitable. Death is certain.

The artist's vision holds yet more ambiguity today. The sporting ducks deliver as well as receive havoc. When they escape the double-barreled shotgun and fly off, they may carry with them nature's revenge, introducing new virus strains right and left: to domestic animals or directly to humans, increasing risks for new pandemics. As we stare into the hunter's barrel in Homer's painting, we could be the sitting ducks.

The connection between the arts and science is not obvious to everyone, though it goes all the way back to the philosophic origins of science (Latin *scientia* = knowledge). The quest for knowledge started with the first humans, who traced their understanding of nature and its creatures on the walls of caves millions of years ago. The quest continued with ancient civilizations, among them the Chinese, who delved seriously into astronomy and healing, the Babylonians and the Egyptians, who collected volumes about nature and its creatures, and the ancient Greek philosophers, who went beyond collecting facts to lay the foundations of natural history and biology. They mastered all then known disciplines: ethics, rhetoric, astronomy, poetics.

Among the greatest thinkers of all time, Aristotle wrote extensively on logic, physics, art, politics, economics, and psychology and made the first serious attempt at classification of animals. In all his treatises, he frequently compared the works of nature with those of art, advocating the superiority of the former. Aristotle was not the last of the era in which nature was the realm of philosophy, but by the time of his death, philosophers had become more concerned with metaphysics and ethics, while the natural sciences fell to other specialists. With the increase of information, establishment of libraries, and invention of the printing press, specialization became the norm, and graduates of higher institutions were given bachelor of arts or bachelor of science degrees. The philosophic origins of science are still implied in the doctor of philosophy degree, though educational systems have largely institutionalized the deep dichotomy between the arts and science, despite their common origins.

In a controversial lecture given at Cambridge University in 1959, British intellectual C. P. Snow (1905–1980) first used the phrase "the two cultures," referring to the world of science and the world of arts to describe their separateness. Snow, who was a physicist, as well as novelist and poet, described his own experiences as a man who frequented both "cultures." "There have been plenty of days when I have spent the working hours with scientists and then gone off at night with some literary colleagues," he wrote, in frustration. "Constantly I felt I was moving among two groups—comparable in intelligence, identical in race, not grossly different in social origin, earning about the same incomes, who have almost ceased to communicate at all, who in intellectual, moral and psychological climate had so little in common, that instead of going from Burlington House of South Kensington to Chelsea, one might have crossed an ocean."

Snow's experiences in 1950s London, likely representative of the thinking of that period elsewhere, seem alive and well in our times. Amidst general enthusiasm about the use of fine art on our journal covers, some readers do question the "gratuitous" use of color by a publication about science, decrying the cost and professing little interest in links to other disciplines. Science reviewers routinely reject Another Dimension manuscripts as "belonging in other venues," even when the science information given in lay terms is sound. And some in the art community are skeptical about links to science. Copyright permission requests for art images to use on the covers of *Emerging Infectious Diseases* have often been rejected by art institutions on the grounds that the art has nothing to do with disease emergence and might be degraded by any association with infection, even if the artists themselves have met untimely deaths from such infections or their community was ravaged by the plagues detailed between the journal covers. "For you can be trained to listen only for the oboe / out of the whole orchestra."[1]

In one of his many portraits, Rembrandt van Rijn painted a *Scholar in His Study*, 1634 (Figure 3), seeking what Aristotle believed all humans naturally desire: knowledge. "Clearly," he wrote in his *Metaphysics*, "it is for no extrinsic advantage that we seek this knowledge . . . since it alone exists for itself." In the old volumes stacked in front of him, the scholar searches for the truth about human existence, suffering, danger, hunger, disease, and survival, knowing that life slips by before the task is done.

Rembrandt himself searched for the truth in the subjects he painted, in the common people whose complexity he sought to capture. And the penetrating analysis and contemplation characteristic of his self-portraits show no less than compulsion to know himself. His work expanded the world of knowledge, for he did not paint semblance alone. He saw, recognized, and expressed inner values and ideas, universal human traits, natural phenomena; explored, understood, and conveyed emotions; and defined, communicated, and commemorated all these. Piece by piece, in individual paintings and collectively in his life's work, he observed and recorded morsels of truth, seeking to understand and capture it.

Whereas his scholar dwelled on words, Rembrandt used color and brushstrokes. For these, along with numbers, notes on the staff, or sheer speculation, are the tools for exploring the universe. And so it goes with science and public health. In isolation like Rembrandt's scholar, in the laboratory or in the field, public health workers search, too, observing, recognizing and meticulously recording relevant information, surveying, delving into the unseen and implied, and expanding knowledge. *Emerging Infectious Diseases* covers seek to bring forth this connection.

Despite continued specialization and a steady drift away from the philosophic origins of science, each era had individual scholars who moved comfortably between multiple seemingly opposing fields. Leonardo da Vinci (1452–1519) was one. Painter, sculptor, musician, architect, anatomist, geologist, botanist, author, he delved into everything from philosophy to mathematics, from warfare to aviation, a field not yet invented in his day. The man who painted *Mona Lisa* wrote about the nervous system: "The frog instantly dies when the spinal cord is pierced. Previous to this it lived without a head, without a heart, or any bowels or intestines or skin. And here,

---

1 From John Stone's "Gaudeamus Igitur: A Valediction."

therefore, it would seem lies the foundation of movement and life." Leonardo believed that it was necessary to master the body's depths to portray its surfaces and professed that painting is a science: "For painting is born of nature, since all visible things were brought forth by nature and these, her children have given birth to painting."

While accomplishment in all disciplines is the gift of genius, the paths to knowledge in individual fields are more egalitarian and accessible. And, fueled by the imagination, compelled by a desire for order, empowered by the ability to see and instinctively recognize the quest for knowledge in any discipline employs certain common elements: observation, recording, perspective. And in science or the arts, multiple perspectives, added dimensions, and adventures in time and space abound.

Part of the brief but brilliant movement known as Renaissance in the North, which included Albert Dürer and Mathias Grünewald, Hans Holbein the Younger was able to grasp and depict the human image in a way that eluded his contemporaries. He was a deliberate observer. In his *Nicholas Kratzer* (Detail), 1528 (Figure 4), it is easy to see how the painter sorted the evidence of physical reality fastidiously gathered for internal character clues. In his portraits, the stubble on the chin or smudge on the thumb was intentional, and the painstaking collection of minute and precise detail built a composite larger than its parts. This intricate composite, much often missed by the casual eye, was purposeful and focused. Free of extraneous or distracting elements, it dispassionately laid out for the viewer a meticulous image to probe for inner meaning and interpretation. Selectively descriptive, proportional, fully cognizant of order and balance, his portraits offered a glimpse into a person's soul and an unadulterated version of the artist's perception of reality.

Observation is equally the domain of science. Fueled by the desire to know, it drives systematic collection of data, the facts needed to formulate a unified concept of nature and the laws that govern it. Scientific observation, like Holbein's artistic equivalent, goes beyond the chaotic collection of facts. Sufficiently ascertained and methodically arranged and analyzed, facts form mathematical models create measurable indicators, predict impact, and calculate costs to produce meaningful and applicable public health models. John Snow's meticulous geospacial maps of cases during the 1854 cholera outbreak in London led to our understanding of the epidemiology of cholera well before its cause was known and culminated in the iconic removal of the Broad Street pump. When graced with clarity of expression, as in Holbein's portraits of distinguished humanists or John Snow's geospatial maps, observation produces good art and good science.

Intrigued by the similarities between the art and physics of the 20th century, British professor Arthur I. Miller wrote *Einstein, Picasso: Space, Time, and the Beauty That Causes Havoc*, a book in which he speculated a connection between the theory of relativity and the modern art movement of cubism. A scientist turned historian-philosopher, Miller investigated whether Einstein and Picasso were working on the same problem, the nature of simultaneity. He found that relativity and cubism were part of a cultural milieu within which both were focused on the nature of time and space and the relation between perception and reality. The purpose of both science and art, Miller noted, is to uncover the reality behind appearances.

"When our first encounter with some object surprises us and we find it novel or very different from what we formerly knew or from what we supposed it ought to be, this causes us to wonder and be astonished at it," wrote 17th-century philosopher René Descartes in his *Passions of the Soul*. Indeed, astonishment awaits anyone who views for the first time the work of Giuseppe Arcimboldi, Milanese painter extraordinaire, portraitist of emperors, and master of illusion.

Arcimboldi's work has been ascribed to mannerism, the art of his times, known for its aesthetic quality, exaggeration, and emphasis on emotion. But his creative imagination moved in an entirely original direction. He turned elements from nature or everyday life into images of his own invention, transforming fruits, vegetables, flowers, animals, or books into enigmatic portraits. The parts were known and clearly understood, but the whole was new and elusive. For these elaborate illusionist tricks or "hieroglyphic wit," poet and theologian Gregorio Comanini called Arcimboldi a "learned Egyptian."

Arcimboldi's *Vertumnus* (1590–1591), which graced one of the covers of *Emerging Infectious Diseases* (Figure 5), was the most famous work of art in Emperor Rudolph II's Prague. In this portrait, the emperor was shown as the Roman god of seasons, gardens, and plants, Vertumnus, who could change at will and was notorious for his disguises. The portrait was eulogized and explicated in a poem by Comanini: "Look at the apple and the peach— / Round, red, and fresh— / That form both cheeks; / Turn your mind to my eyes— / One is a cherry, / The other a red mulberry." Composite creatures have fascinated throughout the ages. Hellenic mythology proposed Chimera, which appeared on pottery 2,500 years ago and was described by Homer in *The Iliad* as "a thing of immortal make, not human, lion-fronted and snake behind, a goat in the middle, and snorting out of breath of the terrible flame of bright fire."

A tempting metaphor, Chimera has been adopted by many civilizations and, more recently, by various disciplines, among them genetics, molecular biology, and virology. Composites abound in nature. Those in the microbial world have gained notoriety in the face of emerging disease, one that Arcimboldi would have delighted in immortalizing. For this complex illusion, instead of fruits or flowers, he would have portrayed MRSA, avian influenza (H5N1), *E. coli* O157: H7, and other hallmarks of emergence: ordinary parts rearranged in a new context. Its specter would have gone beyond astonishment to other common reactions evoked by the master's unpredictable work: unease and foreboding.

After almost two decades of publication, "a time probably between childhood and adolescence in journal years," as Founding Editor Joseph E. McDade put it, *Emerging Infectious Diseases* has not strayed from its goal to communicate effectively the undiminished potential for global emergence of infectious pathogens. Under the enlightened leadership of D. Peter Drotman, physician and art lover, the journal continues to track zoonotic diseases, bacterial pathogenesis, climate change, the role of migratory birds in the spread of West Nile virus, infection in the health care setting, bovine spongiform encephalopathy, the use of anthrax spores in bioterrorism; each theme, a new cover icon. The covers, and stories that accompany them, have evolved, becoming more striking and substantive, thanks to the collaboration and generosity of artists, museums, art foundations, and galleries, who have provided high-quality images and copyright permissions; the *Emerging Infectious Diseases* journal team, who has maximized the effectiveness of cover images and scrutinized the cover stories; authors, who brought to our attention works of art from all over the world; and the many readers, who wrote to encourage our efforts and urge that we continue to bring them the arts with the science.

"For you will learn to see most acutely out of / the corner of your eye / to hear best with your inner ear."[2] How much meaning does cover art bring forth, and how much, if at all, has the blending of the "two cultures" benefited understanding of public health? Would *Emerging Infectious Diseases* be the same without the iconic covers? The value added is not easily ascertained. Yet it would be prudent to continue making the connections. For, as William Carlos Williams put it, "It is difficult / to get the news from poems / yet men die miserably every day / for lack / of what is found there."

Polyxeni Potter
May 2013

Bibliography

Comanini G. *The Figino, or, on the Purpose of Painting: Art Theory in the Late Renaissance.* Maiorino G, Doyle-Anderson A, trans. Toronto, Canada: University of Toronto Press; 2001.

Johns E. *Winslow Homer: The Nature of Observation.* Berkeley, CA: University of California Press; 2002.

Kaufmann TDC. *The Mastery of Nature: Aspects of Art, Science, and Humanism in the Renaissance.* Princeton, NJ: Princeton University Press; 1993.

Potter P. Painting nature on the wing. *Emerg Infect Dis.* 2006;12:180–1.

Myrianthopoulos C. *The philosophic origins of science and the evolution of the two cultures. Emerg Infect Dis.* 2000;6:77–9. Available at: http://wwwnc.cdc.gov/eid/article/6/1/00-0115_article.htm.

Seckel A. *Masters of Deception.* New York, NY: Sterling; 2004.

---

2 John Stone's "Gaudeamus Igitur: A Valediction."

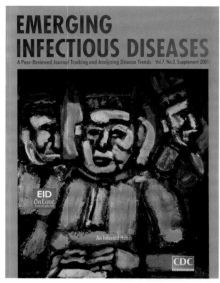

An Infected Heart; http://dx.doi.
org/10.3201/eid0707.AC0707

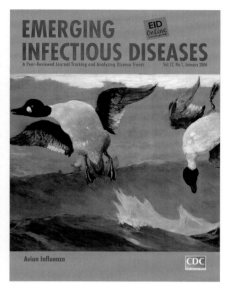

Avian Influenza; http://dx.doi.
org/10.3201/eid1201.AC1201

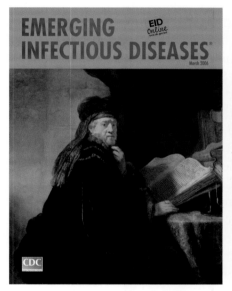

Science, Public Health; http://dx.doi.
org/10.3201/eid1203.AC1203

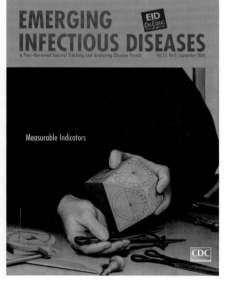

Measurable Indicators; http://dx.doi.
org/10.3201/eid1009.AC1009

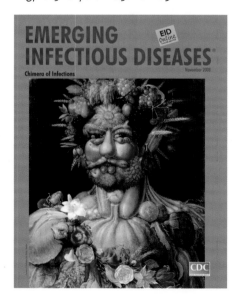

Chimera of Infections; http://dx.doi.
org/10.3201/eid1411.AC1411

Acknowledgments

This book would not have been possible without the support and enthusiasm of D. Peter Drotman, Editor-in-Chief, *Emerging Infectious Diseases*; the collaboration and generosity of the CDC Foundation; Rima Khabbaz, Beth Bell, Ted Pestorius, John O'Connor, Robert W. Pinner, and the National Center for Emerging and Zoonotic Infectious Diseases; Joseph E. McDade, Founding Editor; the late Joshua Lederberg, Robert Shope, and David J. Sencer; Frederick A. Murphy; James M. Hughes; Ruth Berkelman; Anne Schuchat; Stephen M. Ostroff; Brian W.J. Mahy; Kathleen Gensheimer; Pierre and Dominique Rollin; Charles Ben Beard; David Bell; Nina Marano; Martin I. Meltzer; David Morens; J. Glenn Morris; Didier Raoult; David Walker; J. Todd Weber; Kenneth C. Castro; Takeshi Kurata; Charles H. Calisher; John E. McGowan; Robert Swanepoel; Stephen S. Morse; Scott Halstead; David L. Heymann; Judith Aguilar; Nkuchia Mikanatha; Jackie Fox; Judy Gantt; artists, museums, art foundations, and galleries that provided high-quality images; authors, who brought to our attention works of art from all over the world; the *Emerging Infectious Diseases* team: Reginald Tucker, P. Lynne Stockton, Carol Snarey, Tom Gryczan, Anne Mather, Carrie Huntington, Sarah Gregory, Shannon O'Connor, Claudia Chesley, Jean Jones, Karen Foster, Barbara Segal, Tracey Hodges, and Kevin Burlison; CDC scientists and other experts, who provided guidance and encouragement, among them Morris E. Potter, David Swerdlow, and Myron Schultz; Louise Shaw, John Anderton, and Demetri Vacalis; and the many readers, who wrote to encourage our efforts to bring them the arts with the science.

Disease Emergence

B ritish naturalist Langdon W. Smith in his poem "A Tadpole and a Fish" (or "Evolution," 1909) traced events back to the Paleozoic era, the beginning of life. "When you were a tadpole and I was a fish," he told his true love, putting their relationship in perspective, "My heart was rife with the joy of life / for I loved you even then." In his poetic account, Smith expressed eons of evolution, carefully marking landmark events as he went along. "We were Amphibians, scaled and tailed / And drab as a dead man's hand," he noted, "Life by life, and love by love, / We passed through the cycles strange, / And breath by breath, and death by death, / We followed the chain of change." This evolutionary change, so well traced by Smith, is a major factor in the emergence of infections (Fig. T1.1).

The forces that shape emergence are diverse and in constant flux. They come from all areas of life and involve all three aspects of the traditional triangle model of disease causation: host, environment, agent. The forces that promote emergence are therefore genetic and biological, environmental, social, political, and economic. Their convergence supports disease emergence through many factors: microbial adaptation and change; climate, weather, and ecosystems; economic development and land use; human demographics and behavior; technology, industry, travel, and commerce; poverty; and conflict.

The following sections in this collection reflect on factors contributing to disease emergence. Each section contains cover art of *Emerging Infectious Diseases* and essays about the art and how it relates to factors involved in emergence. The final paragraphs in each essay discuss art and science, but the connection between them is intended from the very beginning. It is threaded throughout the essay, by way of the artist's life, the period of the painting and its tensions, and the style of painting, as any of these elements can make an effective connection.

Emergence is fueled by change. Most emerging infections are caused by pathogens present in the environment but brought out of obscurity and given a selective advantage or the opportunity to infect new populations by changing conditions. Pierre-Auguste Renoir's *Luncheon of the Boating Party* opens the section because it exemplifies this notion. Change drives the history of art, too. The impressionist movement, in which Renoir flourished, was a stylistic turn away from academic tradition. It brought artists out of the studio, into the outdoors, to capture an impression, a moment—all that one could ever hope to capture on the canvas.

Other factors in emergence—the way microbes and humans behave, complex interactions in nature, and even developments in biomedical research—can and do feature in the arts. Archibald J. Motley, Jr's *Nightlife* provides the opportunity to

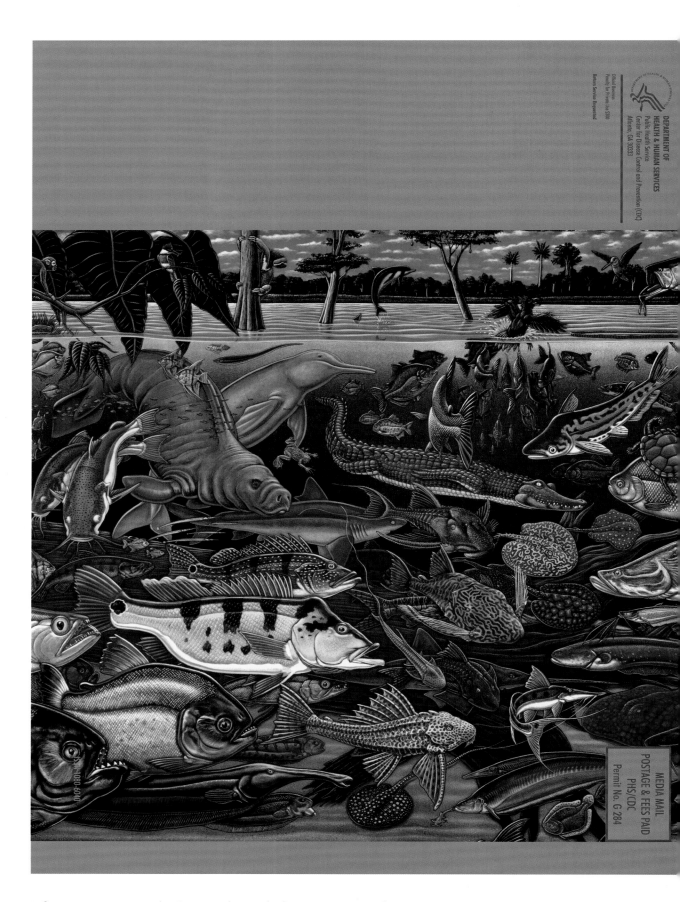

Infectious Diseases in the Amazon; http://dx.doi.org/10.3201/eid1504.AC1504

EMERGING

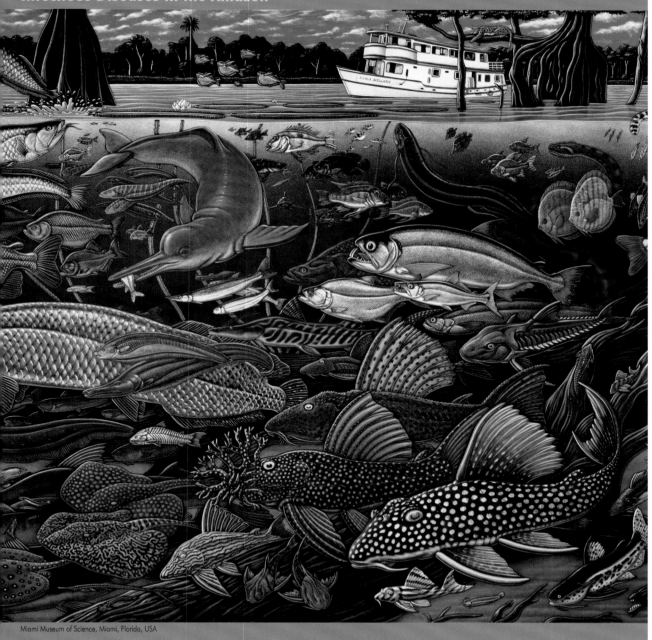

CDC

INFECTIOUS DISEASES®

April 2009

Infectious Diseases in the Amazon

draw a parallel between the spontaneity of the jazz scene flourishing in Chicago's South Side during the 1940s and the group dynamics of microbial populations involved in emergence. Pieter Bruegel the Elder's *Return of the Herd* shows topographical diversity enriched by seasonal cycles and the presence of people and livestock, the perfect backdrop in disease emergence.

Jackson Pollock's *Autumn Rhythm (Number 30)* is a tangle of paths guiding the viewer through the painting itself and through nature as the artist saw it from his back porch in East Hampton. These are not traditional paths, nor do they arrive at the usual destinations. Like paths to scientific discovery, they are often circuitous and surprising, such as a link between an old infection, malaria, and the spread of a new infection, HIV.

Piet Mondrian's *Broadway Boogie Woogie*, with its iconic grid and references to the rhythms of New York City, frames the efforts of artists and scientists to arrive at "true reality." Radical abstraction, a technique mastered by Mondrian in his efforts to get rid of the extraneous and arrive at the essence of things, works well in the laboratory. Michelangelo Merisi da Caravaggio's mellow *Basket of Fruit* is an invitation to discuss disease emergence. The beautiful fruit shows signs of decay, a reminder of the need for vigilance and balance in nature to counter the effects of constant change.

The final piece discussed in this chapter is Leonardo da Vinci's *Mona Lisa*, a classic manifestation of the many connections between arts and science and the embodiment of these connections in the master's own life and work. The enigmatic nature of the portrait rivals the puzzling elements in disease emergence: unknown pathogens, emerging biological threats, ecologic disasters, antimicrobial drug resistance—elements that could benefit from being seen in the context of the arts.

Threading constant changes back and forth, between darkness and light, throughout the eons, with humor and romance, Langdon W. Smith arrived in our times with a reminder about our origins and destiny. "Then as we linger at luncheon here, / O'er many a dainty dish, / Let us drink anew to the time when you / Were a Tadpole and I was a Fish."

Bibliography

Institute of Medicine. *Emerging Infections: Microbial Threats to Health in the United States.* Washington, DC: National Academy Press; 1992.

Potter P. When you were a tadpole and I was a fish. *Emerg Infect Dis.* 2009;15:683–684.

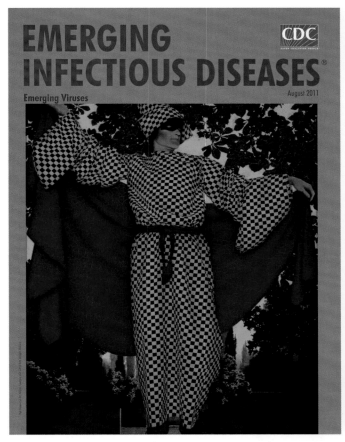

Emerging Viruses; http://dx.doi.org/10.3201/eid1708.AC1708

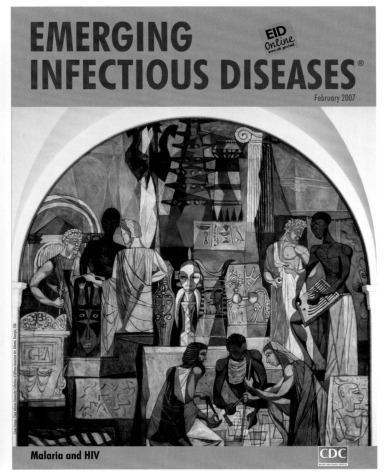

Malaria and HIV; http://dx.doi.org/10.3201/eid1302.AC1302

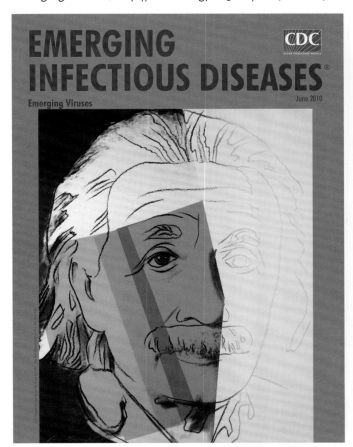

Emerging Viruses; http://dx.doi.org/10.3201/eid1606.AC1606

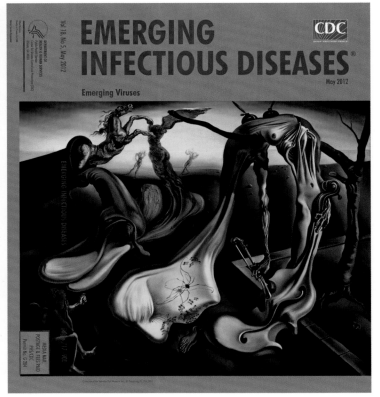

Emerging Viruses; http://dx.doi.org/10.3201/eid1805.AC1805

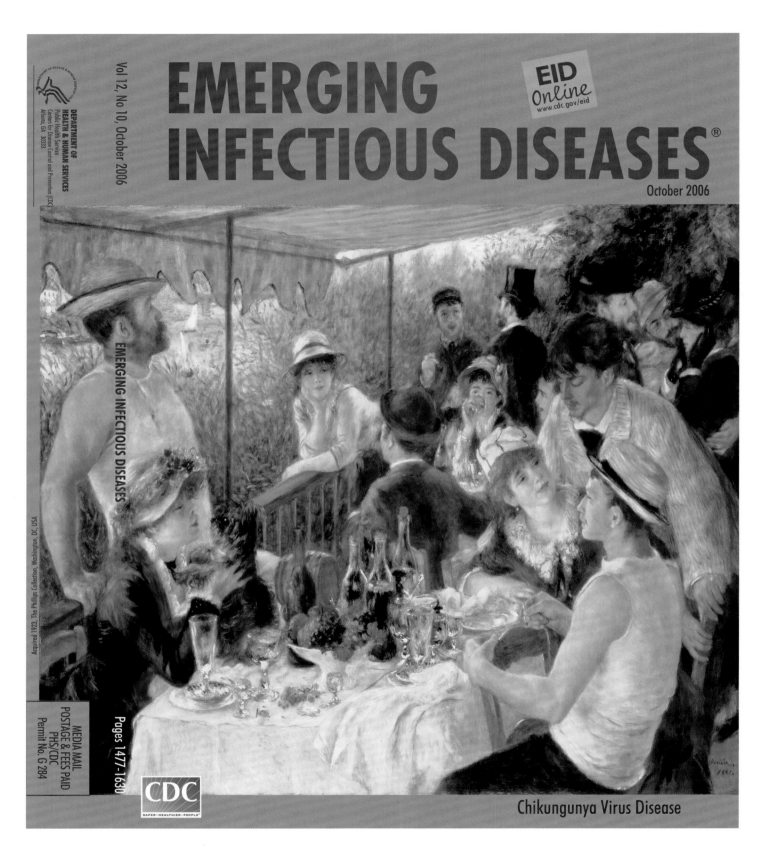

Vol 12, No 10, October 2006

DEPARTMENT OF
HEALTH & HUMAN SERVICES
Public Health Service
Centers for Disease Control and Prevention (CDC)
Atlanta, GA 30333

EMERGING

INFECTIOUS DISEASES®

October 2006

EID
Online
www.cdc.gov/eid

EMERGING INFECTIOUS DISEASES

Acquavella 1923, The Phillips Collection, Washington DC, USA

Pages 1477–1630

MEDIA MAIL
POSTAGE & FEES PAID
PHS/CDC
Permit No. G 284

CDC
SAFER · HEALTHIER · PEOPLE™

Chikungunya Virus Disease

Πάντα ῥεῖ καὶ οὐδὲν μένει [1]

"I'm doing a painting of oarsmen which I've been itching to do for a long time. I'm not getting any younger, and I didn't want to defer this little festivity which later on I won't any longer be able to afford already it's very difficult . . .; one must from time to time attempt things that are beyond one's capacity," wrote Pierre-Auguste Renoir to Paul Bérard, his friend and supporter. The ambitious painting might have been Renoir's response to author and critic Émile Zola's challenge to impressionists in 1880 that, instead of "sketches that are hardly dry," they "create complex paintings of modern life" after "long and thoughtful preparation."

Zola was not alone in challenging artists of his generation. Poet Charles Baudelaire back in 1863 had called for a "painter of modern life," inviting his contemporaries to create art of their own times. Heeding the call, French artists of the late 19th century broke with the past, forging perhaps the most popular movement in the history of art. Radical in their departure from tradition, the impressionists abandoned history as source of inspiration and moved the studio outdoors to capture a moment, an impression, under the changing light of the sun. No longer interested in telling a story, they replaced standard narrative techniques with feathery, interrupted brushstrokes that best described an angle of interest or a fleeting scene of daily life. Their innovations forever changed how art was created and viewed, producing works of unprecedented spontaneity and lightness.

The child of working-class parents, Renoir was born in Limoges, the city in France known for its porcelain and fine china. When he was still young, the family moved to Paris and settled in the Louvre area, where he grew up lighthearted and easygoing in the shadow of the great museum. Despite early affinity for scribbling and drawing, his fine singing voice was noticed first, and he studied under composer Charles Gounod, who encouraged a music career for him. Because of financial constraints, at age 13, he was apprenticed instead to a porcelain painter with the prospect of long-term work at a large factory outside Paris.

At the porcelain shop, his talent for painting was quickly acknowledged, but he continued to paint china, fans, café murals, and window shades, to study in the evenings, and to copy the masters at the Louvre until he could enroll in the École des Beaux-Arts. There, he met Claude Monet, Frédéric Bazille, and Alfred Sisley. The foursome, who shared an aversion to established rules, bonded quickly, painted together, influenced each other, and became founding members of impressionism, along with Paul Cézanne, Edgar Degas, Berthe Morisot, and Camille Pissarro.

"There are no poor people," Renoir believed, denying that lack of means could interfere with happiness, success, or the imagination, even though living expenses and painting supplies were hard to come by for much of his career: "I would several times have given up if Monet had not reassured me with a slap on the back." And when near the end of his life he was invited to the Louvre to view the hanging of one of his works, he mused, "If I had been presented at the Louvre 30 years ago in a wheelchair I would have been shown the door."

---

1 "Everything flows. Nothing stands still" (Herakleitos of Ephesus, c. 2,500 years ago).

Many innovations of this era, among them mixed paints in metal tubes and use of poppy seed oil as binding medium, facilitated the artists' task. And the advent of photography freed them from the need to paint in realistic detail, proposing new ways to focus on subjects. But turmoil brought on by the Franco-Prussian war in 1870 interfered with the full impact of these changes as with the progress of impressionism. Bazille was killed in action; Monet, Pissarro, and Sisley moved to England; and Renoir joined the cuirassiers, though he saw no action.

After the hostilities, Renoir returned to Paris, where he continued to struggle for acceptance. He worked with Monet, painting on the banks of the Seine and the coast of Normandy; traveled to Africa, Spain, and Italy; and by the end of the decade, he had found his own unique voice. His style became more refined and traditional, focusing closely on the human form. "For my part," he freely admitted, "I always defended myself against the charge of being a revolutionary. I always believed and I still believe that I only continued to do what others had done a great deal better before me."

They are "lumpy and obnoxious creatures," wrote the *New York Sun* about Renoir's famed female nudes, exhibited in New York in 1886. Nonetheless, popular success and creature comforts were finally within the artist's reach. He remained extremely prolific (more than 6,000 paintings); despite debilitating arthritis and other health problems, he continued to paint until his death.

No other painting captures Renoir's characteristic joie de vivre and conviviality better than *Luncheon of the Boating Party*. The social ease and camaraderie of his youth seem to have permeated this painting, while gaiety and charm emanate from it toward the viewer, who is tempted to join in. "The picture of rowers by Renoir looks very well," wrote Eugene Manet to his wife, Berthe Morisot. Holiday-making was a favorite theme of the impressionists, who "show their particular talent and attain the summit of their art when they paint our French Sundays . . . kisses in the sun, picnics, complete rest, not a thought about work, unashamed relaxation."

Renoir worked on the complex composition for months, frustrated at times with the unavailability of models, the clustering of figures, the landscape: "I no longer know where I am with it, except that it is annoying me more and more." On this single canvas, he combined still life, genre, landscape, and portraiture to capture food, friends, and conversation near the waterfront. Carefully structured and meticulously finished, this moment at play was to become a cultural icon.

The gathering took place near Chatou, Renoir's favored retreat on the Seine. Once the domain of the affluent, the area now offered pastimes for all. A group of friends assembled on the balcony of the Maison Fournaise. Among them, a historian and art collector, a baron, a poet and critic, a bureaucrat, actresses, and artists Paul Lhote and Gustave Caillebotte, who sat backward in his chair in the right foreground and gazed across the table at Aline Charigot, the young seamstress who later would become Renoir's wife. The youths leaning against the rail are proprietors of the establishment.

"[O]ne cannot imagine these women . . . having been painted by anybody else," wrote art critic Théodore Duret. "They have . . . that graciousness, that roguish charm, which Renoir alone could give to women." Earthy, savvy, and engaging, they light up the scene. The luncheon is finished. The crowd "hangs out" against the clutter of leftover food and drink, gracing the intimate tableau all of us want to be in.

Just beyond the awning, the river flows discreetly in the background. Soon, it will turn dark, the crowd will disperse, the moment will end. The moment and its transient place in constant change, so well understood by the impressionists and masterfully captured by Renoir, have also long puzzled philosophers and scientists and are central to the study of emerging disease. In a world where "everything flows," organisms and their surroundings are constantly changing, and "nothing stands still," vigilance is order of the day. Disease control is as good as the next set of natural circumstances, for as Herakleitos of Ephesus put it 2,500 years ago, "You cannot step twice into the same river, for fresh waters are ever flowing upon you."

Bibliography

Baudelaire C. *Selected Writings on Art and Literature.* New York, NY: Viking Press; 1972.

Centers for Disease Control and Prevention. Claude Monet (1840–1926) Nymphéas (water lilies) 1916–1919. 2002;8:1011.

Davenport G. *Herakleitos and Diogenes.* San Francisco, CA: Grey Fox Press; 1981.

The Great Masters. London, England: Quantum Publishing; 2003.

House J. *Renoir Exhibition Catalog.* London, England: Harry N. Abrams; 1985.

Impressionist Art Gallery. Renoir boating party. Available at: http://www.impressionist-art-gallery.com/renoir_boating_party.html. Accessed August 11, 2006.

The Phillips Collection. Luncheon of the boating party. http://www.phillipscollection.org/html/lbp.html; accessed August 11, 2006.

Renoir A. Luncheon of the boating party. Available at: http://blogs.princeton.edu/wri152-3/s06/mgawrys/auguste_renoir_luncheon_of_the_boating_party.html; accessed August 11, 2006.

Zola E. *Salons.* Geneva, Switzerland: Droz; 1959.

Vol 12, No 2, February 2006

DEPARTMENT OF
HEALTH & HUMAN SERVICES
Public Health Service
Centers for Disease Control and Prevention (CDC)
Atlanta, GA 30333

Official Business
Penalty for Private Use $300

Return Service Requested

EMERGING INFECTIOUS DISEASES®

EID Online
www.cdc.gov/eid

February 2006

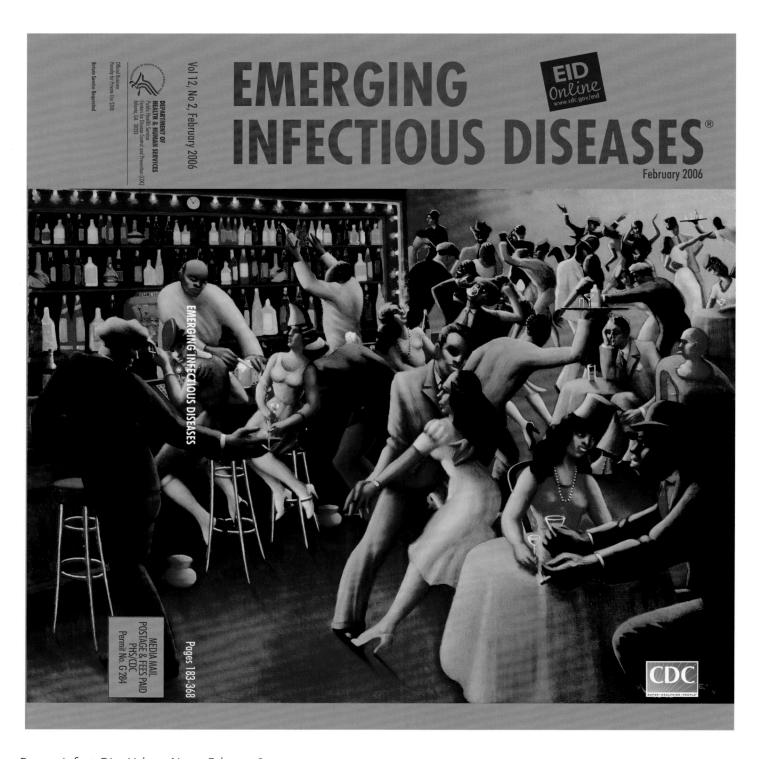

EMERGING INFECTIOUS DISEASES

Pages 183–368

MEDIA MAIL
POSTAGE & FEES PAID
PHS/CDC
Permit No. G 284

CDC

Emerg. Infect. Dis., Vol. 12, No. 2, Feb. 2006

HOST-PATHOGEN-VENUE COMBINATIONS
AND ALL THAT JAZZ

"To call yourself a New Yorker you must have been to Harlem at least once. Every up-to-date person knows Harlem, and knowing Harlem generally means that one has visited a night club or two," wrote novelist and editor Wallace Thurman. "The music is good, the dancers are gay, and setting is conducive to joy." In the 1920s, nightclubs, bars, and cabarets were much in vogue in most of the Western world. In New York, many talented entertainers worked in these clubs—Duke Ellington's orchestra, Cab Calloway's band, Lena Horne, Adelaide Hall. Chicago became a jazz center with more than 100 clubs. "Midnight was like day," wrote poet Langston Hughes describing the city's South Side. The exotic, glamorous, intoxicated environment of these clubs, which dominated American entertainment for most of the 20th century, was a main source of inspiration to Chicago painter Archibald Motley.

Motley was born in New Orleans, Louisiana, but his family moved north when he was very young. His mother was a schoolteacher, his father a railroad man, operating a buffet car running on the Michigan Central. Even as a child he sketched scenes and people around him and knew that he wanted to be an artist. The elder Motley mentioned his son's ambitions to Frank W. Gunsaulus of the Armour Institute, a train patron, who paid the youth's first year's tuition at the Art Institute of Chicago. A receptive and eager student, Motley studied under accomplished painter Karl Buehr, who encouraged and advised him: "I want to tell you something, Mr. Motley. I don't want you to ever change your style of painting . . . please continue it, for my sake."

At the Art Institute, Motley indulged his admiration of the Old Masters, particularly Dutch painter Frans Hals, and was exposed to the work of other American artists (George Bellows, John Sloan, Randall Davey). His graduation in 1918 coincided with the advent of the Harlem Renaissance, a cultural movement encompassing the literary, musical, visual, and performing arts and promoting celebration of African identity and heritage. Motley exhibited widely and received many prestigious awards, among them a John Simon Guggenheim Fellowship, which gave him the opportunity to live in Paris for a year. "It is remarkable and beautiful . . . the way the light travels on the pigmentation of the skin, how gradually the light changes from warm into cool in various faces. . . . I used to go to the Louvre and study, oh, I studied Delacroix, I studied all the old masters carefully. You know, what we call 'in' painting, the passages of tones."

Motley was very productive in Paris. He completed 12 paintings, among them the celebrated *Blues*, inspired by the local nightclub scene. But he returned to Chicago to exhibit the work. "Artists feel that they're more readily recognized in Europe than they are here in America. . . . I am staying here in wonderful America. And I love Chicago."

"I think that every picture should tell a story," Motley noted. His narrative paintings, like the work of Frans Hals, peered into the lives of the common people, whom he painted with enthusiasm. But while 17th-century Dutch masters ridiculed drunkenness and warned against the moral laxity of the tavern scene, he viewed social life with affection and offered a glittering rendition of people at play.

The club scene with its "total experience" setting provided a perfect backdrop. Extravagantly decorated rooms filled with smoke and spirits called for people to dress up and step out, to escape the reality of postwar depression and social inequity and experience fantasy and luxury in an electrified, unreal environment. His empathetic portraits and earthy descriptions reflected both his own exuberant love of life and the nightclub scene's whole new view of celebrating: good food, music and dance, and the chance to see and be seen.

"When my grandmother found out that I was playing jazz music," said jazz composer Jelly Roll Morton, "she told me that I had disgraced the family and forbade me to live in the house." The music played inside colorful, thickly populated nightclubs all over the United States and spreading around the world, cool jazz, red hot jazz, all manner of jazz, was not always viewed as art form. The music's irregular, sensuous tunes, mixing folk with blues, engaging new instruments, embracing regional sounds, evolved independently in many locations and created an incredible diversity of sounds and styles.

Nightlife, on this month's cover, one of Motley's most celebrated works, is a glimpse of the action at a dance hall in Chicago's Bronzeville neighborhood. Painted during World War II, the picture does not address the dire global circumstances. It focuses instead on a lighthearted moment of gaiety, inside a comfortable establishment, vibrant with the sounds of music, dancing, and conversation. A lively jazz band in the background guides the figures. Diagonal lines indicate sharp syncopated movement amidst free-flowing activity around the dance floor.

The stage is framed with bar paraphernalia, stools, and tables. But the scene is not about the venue. The artist is painting energy and motion, the group dynamic of a community, laughing, gesturing, mingling. The figures are bold but stylized, so the viewer is not distracted by individual features. Body language and overall carriage are harmonious and integrated, and the crowd is engaged and receptive.

Even as Motley focused on the moment's thrill inside a nightclub, he created a microcosm analogous to broader outside reality, an allegory of the world. The stylish crowd socializing and the jazz band orchestrating their movements mirror the group dynamics of microbial populations, swinging to nature's tune in niches they make for themselves. The spontaneity of jazz music and its adaptations to local culture over time around the globe parallel the emergence and export of new diseases from their seedbeds to audiences the world over. A glance at this issue's contents confirms the immense diversity of disease emergence over time and place, from birds with flu and *Helicobacter* infections to drug-resistant HIV strains, from Nipah virus to *Arcobacter*, from dengue to ameba-associated pneumonia. All neatly choreographed to music we cannot yet hear.

Bibliography

Oral history interview with Archibald Motley, 1978 Jan. 23-1979 Mar. 1. Available at http://www.aaa.si.edu/collections/oralhistories/transcripts/motley78.htm. Accessed April 24, 2013.

Culture Shock. The devil's music, 1920s jazz. Available at: http://www.pbs.org/wgbh/cultureshock/beyond/jazz.html. Accessed April 24, 2013.

Thurman W. *Negro Life in New York's Harlem*. Girard, KS: Haldeman-Julius Company; 1928.

EMERGING
INFECTIOUS DISEASES®

EID
Online
www.cdc.gov/eid

November 2007

CDC
SAFER · HEALTHIER · PEOPLE™

Landscape of Emerging Infections

THE PANORAMIC LANDSCAPE OF HUMAN SUFFERING

The Old Masters were never wrong about suffering, wrote W. H. Auden. They understood how it takes place, "While someone else is eating or opening a window or just walking dully along." Auden was referring to the work of Pieter Bruegel the Elder, which dwelled on suffering, along with labor and merrymaking, the lot of simple folk. He painted them with such dedication it earned him the title "Peasant Bruegel."

He so delighted in the behavior of peasants, he disguised himself as one, and went out into the countryside to mingle with them during their feasts and weddings; he "brought gifts like the other guests, claiming relationship or kinship with the bride or groom." He observed "how they ate, drank, danced, capered, or made love, all of which he was well able to reproduce cleverly and pleasantly," wrote chronicler Karel van Mander, "men and women of the Campine and elsewhere—naturally, as they really were." So well did he represent them and through them all of humanity, that in the words of his friend the famed cartographer Abraham Ortelius, "he painted many things that cannot be painted."

He was held in high esteem by scholars of his day, among them poet and engraver Dierick Volckherzoon Coornhert, who once was so impressed by Bruegel's work, he wrote, "I examined it with pleasure and admiration from top to bottom for the artistry of its drawing and the care of the engraving . . . methinks I heard moaning, groaning and screaming and the splashing of tears in this portrayal of sorrow."

What we know about the artist comes from Karel van Mander's *Painter's Book*, published in 1604, some 35 years after Bruegel's death. He was likely born in the late 1520s in Breda (modern Netherlands); lived and worked in Antwerp and Brussels; and apprenticed with sculptor, architect, painter, designer of tapestry and stained glass Pieter Coecke van Aelst, whose daughter he later married. The apprenticeship had little influence on his style but did introduce him to humanist circles and the work of Maria Verhulst Bessemers, his mother-in-law, a skilled miniaturist and illuminator who experimented with tempera on linen.

After 1559, he dropped the "h" from his name, though his sons, Jan and Pieter the Younger, retained the original Brueghel spelling. Too young at the time of his death to learn from their father, the sons studied with their grandmother and became important artists in their own right, part of a brilliant legacy of four generations in the 16th and 17th centuries.

Like many northern artists, Bruegel traveled to Italy. He visited Naples and Messina and lived in Rome, where he worked with Giulio Clovio, the "prince of miniaturists" according to Giorgio Vasari. Inspired by Italian landscape painting, he "did many views from nature so it was said of him when he traveled through the Alps that he had swallowed all the mountains and rocks and spat them out again, after his return, onto his canvases and panels, so closely was he able to follow nature there and in his other works."

Drawings of the Alpine landscape published as engravings when he returned to Antwerp brought him early fame. They were completed during his long association as draftsman for leading print publisher Hieronymus Cock. Along with drawing and designing for Cock's engravings, Bruegel continued to paint. He favored multifigure compositions in which groups were seen from above. Some of his paintings recalled the fantastic landscapes of the ever popular Hieronymus Bosch (c. 1450–1516). So successful was the resemblance that humanist Domenicus Lampsonius complimented Bruegel by calling him "a second Bosch." But the Master's interest in the burlesque was brief.

Bruegel came to landscape painting from the tradition of Joachim Patinir and the Netherlandish painters, inventors of the genre, and from the Venetians, whose work so impressed him. But his genius went far beyond these. His compositions, carefully structured and realistic, were spare, ahead of their time in their focus on shape and movement. Intrigued by the workings of nature, he turned away from idealized landscapes. Familiar with the common people, he translated moralizing and proverbial tales into vernacular earthy scenes infused with humor and whimsy. "There was always more than he painted."

Landscape painting has been linked to the rise of Antwerp. The city on the Schelde was a prosperous commercial and publishing center. Demand for luxury goods created a flourishing art market, for as Karel van Mander put it, "art gladly resides with wealth." Antwerp's guild, in which Bruegel was accepted as Master, boasted 300 artists, at a time when the city supported 169 bakers, 78 butchers, and 75 fishmongers. Landscapes were painted for the open market, and prints were big business.

Unlike many of his contemporaries who struggled to compete, Bruegel was patronized by connoisseurs and earned fame and prestige during his lifetime. Wealthy merchant Niclaes Jongelinck owned 16 of his works. On commission, Bruegel painted for Jongelinck's home a series representing the seasons. Five of likely six panels survive, among them, *Return of the Herd*, on this month's cover. Though created in the medieval tradition of calendar scenes, each panel focused not on the labors of the season alone but on the transformations of nature and its interrelationships with humans.

The Seasons represents the mature work of a man called by his contemporaries "the most perfect artist of the century" and contains many innovations used to express weather conditions, light effects, and human behavior. Symbolic color was used to invoke seasonal atmosphere. Precise execution gave way to faster, sketchier, more spontaneous technique, allowing greater naturalness and expression in the figures. Paint was thinner to let underpaint show. Peter Paul Rubens later studied this technique. *Return of the Herd* has a circular rhythm linking the foreground with the background, the ritual return of the herd with mountains and gathering clouds. The high-horizon vista of trees, running water, and hills dominates. Yet, tempered by the presence of unvarnished humanity, the cosmographic vision turns parochial. Winter is just around the corner. Humans and animals head for cover. "Nature herself feared being outdone by Bruegel." But his fertile metaphorical terrain, with its rich tonal variations, rhythmical movement, and insuppressible aura of death and regeneration, without parallel in the 16th century, may have found its match in our times. The landscape of emerging infections, broad, diverse, and fueled by human activity, rivals Bruegel's in geographic expanse, topographical detail, and the threat of unrelenting human hazard: antimicrobial drug resistance, violent conflict, HIV/AIDS, vectorborne infections, epizootic (H5N1) and pandemic flu, ecologic disasters, and community- and hospital-acquired infections. Human suffering, as Auden put it, so well understood by the Old Masters, continues unabated, "in a corner, / some untidy spot / where the dogs go on with their doggy life and the torturer's horse / scratches its innocent behind on a tree."

Bibliography

Büttner N. *Landscape Painting*. New York, NY: Abbeville Press Publishers; 2006.
The Great Masters. London, England: Quantum Publishing; 2003.

ONENESS, COMPLEXITY, AND THE DISTRIBUTION
OF DISEASE

"On the floor," said Jackson Pollock, "I feel more at ease. I feel nearer, more a part of the painting . . . I can walk around it, work from the four sides and literally be in the painting . . . akin to the . . . Indian sand painters of the West." Immediacy to the artwork is hallmark of abstract expressionism or the New York School, a revolutionary art movement that shifted the center of artistic avant-garde from Europe to the United States. Born in the aftermath of World War II, this movement valued the inner world over external objects and articulated an emotional landscape fraught with uncertainty and despair.

"Modern art to me is nothing more than the expression of contemporary aims of the age that we're living in," Pollock wrote. The age was the postwar period, filled with anxiety, shocked by the atom bomb, changed by machines, immersed in Freudian theory and psychoanalysis, swinging with improvisational jazz. To this age, Pollock brought abstraction suited to his radical prototype, volatile personality, roughness, and impatience. Along with Willem De Kooning, Barnett Newman, Mark Rothko, and others, he elevated the act of painting, advocating that it should be as direct and fundamental as what it was trying to express and that it could, itself, promote emotional expression.

"I continue to get further away from the usual painter's tools such as easel, palette, brushes. . . . I prefer sticks, trowels, knives and dripping fluid paint or a heavy impasto with sand, broken glass," said Pollock about his expressive technique, which came to be known as action painting. The need to make an original statement, always at the heart of artistic and other human endeavor, permeated not only the subject matter of abstract expressionism but also its technical execution. Well versed in the language of art, he knew and admired the work of Picasso, the surrealists, and Mexican muralists and experimented with several styles, seeking a new idiom.

"I shall be an Artist of some kind. If nothing else I shall always study the Arts," wrote Pollock as a young man. He was born in Cody, Wyoming, the youngest of five children and migrated with his family to Arizona and California, where he studied art at Manual Arts High School in Los Angeles. At 18, he moved to New York City, settled in Greenwich Village, and enrolled in the Art Students League, where he studied with American regionalist painter Thomas Hart Benton, later his mentor and friend.

"Thank you, but not so hard, not so hard," he admonished a colleague who hit him in frustration. Pollock was known to use his artist's hands in anger. He was excitable, contentious, and mistrustful of authority. He got in fights and more than once slugged his instructors in school. Those who knew him in his early years thought he could not draw. As an adult, he struggled with creative blocks, depression, and alcoholism and was torn with self-doubt. Two of his brothers, who lived with him in Manhattan, encouraged him to seek psychoanalysis, thinking that if he could "hold himself together," his work would become "of real significance," because his painting was "abstract, intense, evocative." Jungian psychoanalysis, particularly the conflict between reason and the unconscious, made Pollock aware of how central his emotions had become in his life and work.

DEPARTMENT OF
HEALTH & HUMAN SERVICES
Public Health Service
Centers for Disease Control and Prevention (CDC)
Atlanta, GA 30333

Official Business
Penalty for Private Use $300

Return Service Requested

Malaria and HIV

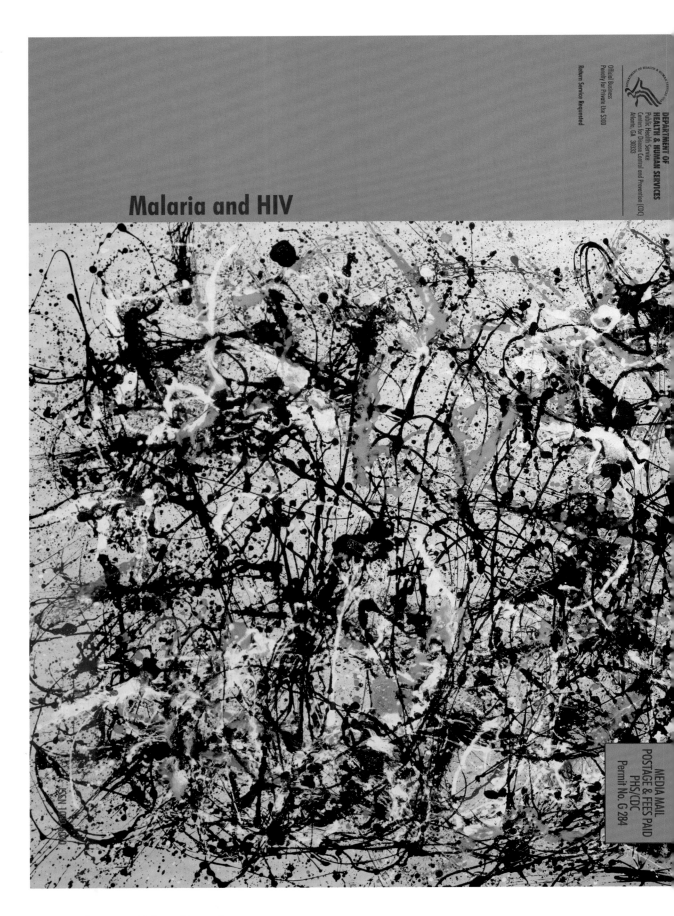

ISSN 1080-6040

MEDIA MAIL
POSTAGE & FEES PAID
PHS/CDC
Permit No. G-284

EMERGING
INFECTIOUS DISEASES

EID Online
www.cdc.gov/eid

A Peer-Reviewed Journal Tracking and Analyzing Disease Trends   Vol.11, No.9, September 2005

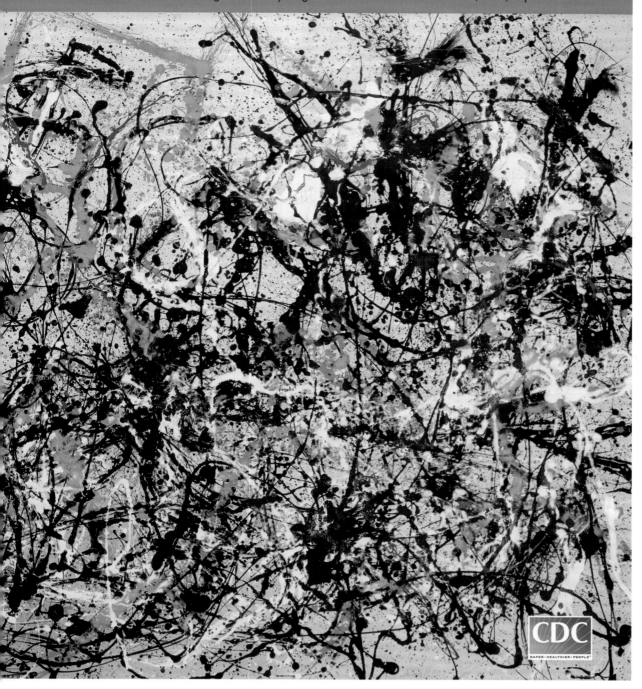

CDC
SAFER·HEALTHIER·PEOPLE™

In 1943, Pollock's work attracted the attention of Peggy Guggenheim, influential art dealer and patron, who commissioned a large mural. He tore down the walls of his Greenwich apartment to accommodate the huge canvas and completed the painting in a marathon 15 hours. In 1945, he left the city for East Hampton, Long Island. There in the countryside and away from distractions, he did his most innovative work. He died at age 44 of injuries in a car wreck, not knowing what he had accomplished or could have accomplished in a full life span.

"The modern artist is working with space and time and expressing his feelings rather than illustrating," Pollock believed. For hours he sat on the back porch of his farmhouse, taking in the natural environment, absorbing its shapes and complexity, which would later find their way into his thick interwoven designs. His studio, a converted barn, allowed space for large yachting canvases he bought at a nearby hardware store. He invented a new way to apply paint, one that combined maximum spontaneity with rigid control and produced images unprecedented in the history of art. "Dancing" on the spread canvas, Pollock created on its surface spontaneous images shaped by the trajectory of his motions. He controlled, adjusted, and modified color and shapes in paintings that were continuous, complex, and provocative and contained none of the traditional elements of composition—perspective, balance, borders, beginning, end.

"Is this a painting? Is this a painting?" he agonized. Not alone in his bewilderment, the artist was torn between marveling at and doubting his creation. "Jack the dripper," he was dubbed by the critics, who knew not what to make of these awesome tangles of paint. Was he making a profound statement or "flinging paint in the public's face?" *Autumn Rhythm* is characteristic of Pollock's most mature work. The painting contains no illusion of physical space or shapes, only textured color and seemingly unrelated lines. Reaction can only come from what the viewer feels or sees in the painting, from the striations of color and texture, which come to life as the eye moves from web cluster to color mass, discovering depth in flat surfaces, relationships in unconnected lines, muted softness, deep darkness, a delicate weave of lines, dots, swirls, and curves, overlapping into a labyrinth of infinite possibilities.

"I am nature," Pollock asserted. Through his creative "dance" he saw himself as one, not only with the painting but with its subject as well. By pouring a constant stream of paint directly out of a can, he produced a continuous trajectory, a web of crisscrossing trajectories, filled with energy and motion and reminiscent of organic shapes, trees, woods, designs of increasing complexity—nature's fingerprint as seen from his back porch in East Hampton.

Viewing *Autumn Rhythm* is a personal experience, one shared with Pollock in his moment of inspiration. Caught in the colorful web, we follow the infinite enamel skeins until the complex interconnections levitate off the canvas and we become part of the web.

The oneness and complexity of Pollock's paintings, his spontaneous dance to the rhythm of nature and the riddles of the inner world, speak to the biomedical scientist in a direct and fundamental way. For, in science as in art, entangled trails lead to unanticipated discoveries.

Disease distribution follows the complex, repetitive, and cumulative patterns of nature. Like Pollock's creations, it traverses spontaneous routes and arrives at unpredictable destinations. In some infectious diseases, malaria for one, incidence and spread have been defined by environmental factors: rainfall, temperature, elevation, and distribution of vector mosquitoes. Emergence of HIV unveiled additional interconnections as it inflated immunocompromised populations. No longer defined by vector distribution alone but now linked to distribution of HIV, malaria cases and deaths have increased, turning an old scourge and a new one into unlikely partners.

Bibliography

Jackson Pollock. http://naples.cc.stonybrook.edu; accessed June 27, 2005.

Johnson EH, ed. *American Artists on Art from 1940–1980.* New York, NY: Harper and Row; 1982.

Koppelman D. Jackson Pollock and true and false ambition: the urgent difference. Available at: http://www.terraingallery.org/Jackson-Pollock-Ambition-DK.html. Accessed April 25, 2013.

Korenromp EL, Williams BG, de Vlas SJ, et al. Malaria attributable to the HIV-1 epidemic, sub-Saharan Africa. *Emerg Infect Dis.* 2005;11:1412–1410-1419

Mathews HV. Pollock in perspective. Available at: http://www.frontlineonnet.com/fl1614/16140700.htm. Accessed April 25, 2013.

PBS Newshour. Jackson Pollock. Available at: http://www.pbs.org/newshour/bb/entertainment/jan-june99/pollock_1-11.html. Accessed April 25, 2013.

Taylor RP, Spehar B, Clifford CW, Newell BR. The visual complexity of Pollock's dripped fractals. Available at: http://materialscience.uoregon.edu/taylor/art/TaylorICCS2002.pdf. Accessed June 1, 2005.

EMERGING
INFECTIOUS DISEASES

EID Online
www.cdc.gov/eid

A Peer-Reviewed Journal Tracking and Analyzing Disease Trends   Vol.10, No.10, October 2004

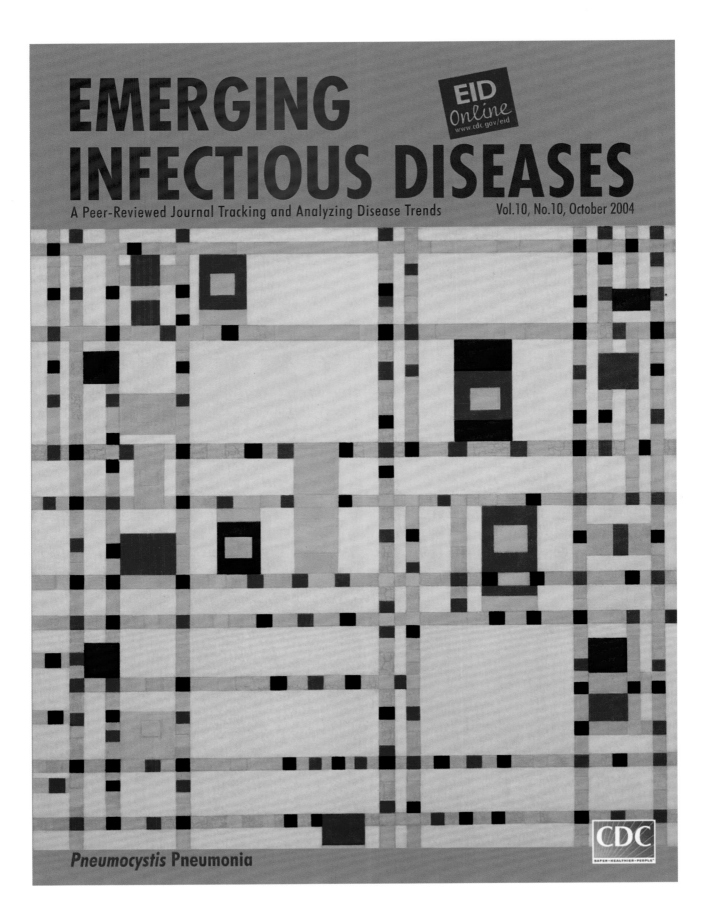

Pneumocystis Pneumonia

CDC
SAFER·HEALTHIER·PEOPLE

MOLECULAR TECHNIQUES AND THE TRUE CONTENT OF REALITY

"Everything was spotless white, like a laboratory. In a light smock, with his clean-shaven face, taciturn, wearing heavy glasses, Mondrian seemed more a scientist or priest than an artist. The only relief to all the white were large matboards, rectangles in yellow, red and blue, hung in asymmetric arrangements on all the walls." This description of Piet Mondrian's New York studio sheds light on the man who went beyond all efforts of his generation to achieve abstraction in search of absolute reality.

Mondrian's incongruous appearance and even his name (changed from Mondriaan) reflected his transformation during an artistic career that spanned two world wars. Over the 20 years during which he studied abstraction, he steadily moved toward simplicity and purity. He abandoned all that was representational, turning himself from a painter of landscapes and flowers to one that tolerated only horizontal and vertical lines, flat surfaces, and primary colors. Forging a style that was in its essence mathematical, he selected single motifs and worked on them until they were completely stripped of form and reduced to lines or grids: "I saw the ocean as a series of pluses and minuses."

Mondrian was born into a family of artists in Amersfoort, Holland, and was brought up a Calvinist. His early work, mostly landscapes of the Dutch countryside, bespoke the realism featured in his academic training and a sense of order and surface geometry reminiscent of Jan Steen. Influenced by the work of Vincent van Gogh and an interest in theosophy, his paintings became increasingly abstract.

Theosophy, a philosophic movement of the late 19th century that focused on the spiritual structure of the universe, also influenced the work of Wassily Kandinsky, Kazimer Malevich, and other contemporaries. Mondrian traveled to Paris, where he met Georges Braque and other leading artists and was exposed to the abstracting qualities of cubism and the primary colors of fauvism. His work in Paris culminated in a new art movement known as De Stijl or neoplasticism.

The term *neoplasticism* was coined by Mondrian's friend the Dutch mathematician and theosophist M. J. H. Schoenmaekers. "Plastic" referred to a formal structure underlying everything in nature. In abstract art, distracting elements around this fundamental structure were removed, leaving fragments of objects or, in Mondrian's work, black bands and color rectangles. The challenge was to find, out of infinite possibilities, the right relation between these bands and the rectangles they formed.

Establishing the right relation between line and color (band and rectangle) was the path to "pure reality," which Mondrian defined as equilibrium "through the balance of unequal but equivalent oppositions." Not a single line or color could be moved without disrupting this balance. "The rhythm of relations of color and size," he wrote in *Natural Reality and Abstract Reality*, "makes the absolute appear in the relativity of time and space." Mondrian's principles of rigorous abstraction, refined geometry, and exquisite nonsymmetrical balance have influenced modern architectural, industrial, and other nonfigurative design.

When Mondrian arrived in New York during World War II, he was 70 years old and in poor health, yet his creativity reached a new height before his death of pneumonia in 1944. *Broadway Boogie Woogie* was the last painting he finished. Born of sheer fascination with the vital culture of 1940s New York, this celebrated work seems to synthesize the elements of his artistic philosophy. As if finally confident in the sound structural relations between bands and rectangles of color, Mondrian made one more radical abstraction. Modifying his hallmark black grid, he integrated bands and color in a series of small, unequal but equivalent rectangles. The result seems an exuberant abstraction of New York itself, a fluorescent skeleton of its architectural blocks, the rhythm of its heartbeat, the lights of its nightlife on an infinite flickering marquis.

A lover of music and dance, Mondrian was in tune with the culture of his day. He clearly knew boogie-woogie, the dynamic, colorful music that reached its peak in 1938, when Albert Ammons, Pet Johnson, and Meade Lux Lewis brought it to Carnegie Hall. The repetitive eight-to-the-bar bass line of boogie-woogie blues structure found a perfect home in Mondrian's disciplined rectangles. Yellow, red, blue, gray, white boxes, aligned in regular intervals and punctuated by improvised riffs, form a seamless, perfectly balanced grid. Brimming with joyous movement and effortless rhythm, a parade of blinking steps engages the viewer in an ingenious visual dance.

The equilibrium Mondrian sensed in the universe and sought in radical abstraction is well known to biologists. Modern molecular techniques, stripping organisms of all but their genetic base, array clumped fragments—DNA fingerprints—the biologist's version of Mondrian's grid. The fragments, used to type and characterize agents such as *Pneumocystis jirovecii*, causative agent of *Pneumocystis* pneumonia, provide scientists a glimpse of pure reality, along with information on sources of infection, patterns of transmission, and potential emergence of antimicrobial resistance.

Bibliography

Boogie woogie piano: from Barrelhouse to Carnegie Hall. Available at: http://colindavey.com/BoogieWoogie/articles/ofamart.htm. Accessed August 31, 2004.

Beard CB, Roux P, Nevez G, et al. Strain typing methods and molecular epidemiology of *Pneumocystis* pneumonia. *Emerg Infect Dis.* 2004;10:1729–1735.

Hall K. Theosophy and the emergence of modern abstract art. Available at: https://www.theosophical.org/publications/1446. Accessed April 27, 2013.

Mondrian P. Natural reality and abstract reality. Available at: http://www.neiu.edu/~wbsieger/Art319/319Read/319Mondrian.pdf. Accessed June 4, 2013.

Sylvester D. *About Modern Art.* New York, NY: Henry Holt & Co; 1997.

Zuffi S. *One Thousand Years of Painting.* Spain: Borders Press; 2001.

EMERGING
INFECTIOUS DISEASES

EID
Online
www.cdc.gov/eid

A Peer-Reviewed Journal Tracking and Analyzing Disease Trends   Vol.9, No.12, December 2003

CDC
SAFER · HEALTHIER · PEOPLE

Disease emergence and control

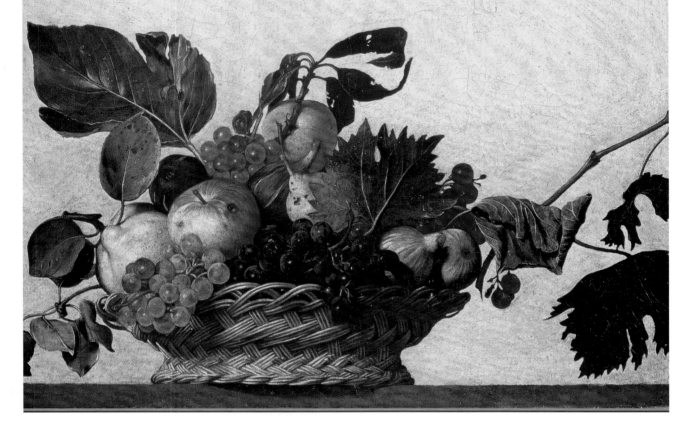

CHIAROSCURO IN ART AND NATURE

Born Michelangelo Merisi, Caravaggio was later renamed after his hometown in northern Italy, a practice not unusual in his day. His father, an architect and major-domo to the Marquis of Caravaggio, died of the plague when the artist was still young, leaving him under the protection of the art-loving marquis. Like many children of his day, he learned early how to grind pigments for painting, and soon he was apprenticed to a good studio in Milan. At 21, he moved to Rome, anxious, if not fully qualified, to compete in the capital's bustling art world. This move to Rome began the tumultuous life journey of a man who changed the art of his day, had many followers (the Caravaggisti), and influenced future masters, from Rembrandt to Velázquez.

In Rome's cosmopolitan art scene, the young Caravaggio found scant opportunity and slow recognition. Handicapped by his exuberance, fiery temper, and heightened artistic sensitivity, he was unable to cope with restrictions and authority. Brash, overbearing, and irascible, he became entangled in riotous brawls and walked the disorderly side of the capital. All the while, he painted mellow canvases overflowing with empathy, humanity, and compassion. Inventing a new, radical kind of realism, he populated his pictures with ordinary people, embracing their imperfections and weaknesses with a candor that many of his contemporaries mistook for vulgarity.

As if to decipher the contradictions and paradoxes of his own shadowy character, Caravaggio explored the interplay of light and dark, known in Italian as chiaroscuro. In an exaggerated theatrical style, he cast light selectively, adding drama to scenes, illuminating figures, and creating a poetic reality that was both earthy and mystical.

With remarkable immediacy, he painted potent images of beheadings and executions, perhaps anticipating the horror of his own punishment for unsavory behavior, not the least of which was killing his opponent during a tennis game. Arrested, imprisoned, pardoned, and constantly on the edge, Caravaggio continued to paint while living in exile for 4 years. The disregard for limits that distinguished his work dominated his life and in the end overcame his artistic promise. Injured during one final, ironically mistaken, arrest, and feverish with malaria, he died before age 40.

During the early days of his tenure in Rome, unknown, unemployed, and unappreciated, Caravaggio painted religious images and baskets of fruit and flowers. Still-life painting, the domain of beginners since antiquity, ranked low on the hierarchical order of pictorial genres. Reduced to it by circumstance, Caravaggio elevated the genre to new heights, creating a European tradition that explored the "secret lives of objects."

"I put as much effort in painting a basket of flowers as I do in painting human figures," Caravaggio told an early patron. In an innovative move toward abstraction, he allowed objects (their form, angle, solidity, composition) to define space. Instead of idealizing them, as the classicists advocated, he painted their imperfections, investing them with uniqueness and content. And instead of centering compositions on the canvas, he thrust them provocatively in the viewer's face, demanding attention and participation.

"I would have . . . hung a similar basket next to it but as no one was able to attain its incomparable beauty and excellence, it remained alone," 17th-century cardinal Federico Borromeo said of Caravaggio's *Basket of Fruit*.

This "incomparable" basket, probably painted over a number of days, has a weathered familiarity, its ripened contents settled, its branches jutting stiffly out the edge. Though representing tradition and plentitude, the fruit is past its prime. Only the tart quince seems to be holding firm. Soft and lusterless, the apple is pockmarked and flawed. The grapes hang heavy, their translucent skin spotted and brown against the plump figs. The leaves, colors fading, edges curling and snarled, are brittle and crinkly. Yet, against an abstract backdrop of brilliant gold leaf, this laden basket exudes comfortable elegance, tangible beauty, graceful maturity.

Caravaggio's painting is not just a lyrical composition of forms. Engaging the senses in virtual abundance, which like life itself is all too ephemeral, the basket comments on the complexity and vanity of nature. Defying the moment of creation, the diverse image spans instead the life of the fruit, reflecting on its inevitable decay. The blemishes, intentional and central to the theme, are not brought on by precipitous mishap but by nature. Uncontrolled environment (temperature, moisture, microorganisms) has disrupted the fruit's normal physiology, devitalizing the skin, allowing invasion of pathogens, and promoting decomposition.

In our world, as in Caravaggio's, where light and darkness, beauty and horror, engagement and danger are constantly at play, survival depends on keeping the elements of nature in balance, constantly tracking their course, monitoring their moves, and checking their excesses. Left untended and uncontrolled, nature's elements will thrive to unfair advantage, mutate to our detriment, and travel to our doorstep. In Mongolia, Vietnam, and other formerly out-of-the-way places, where control efforts have not always kept pace, old scourges (tuberculosis, brucellosis, plague, tularemia) maintain their insidious hold, a blemish on world health and a threat to balance and control.

Bibliography

Christiansen K. Caravaggio (Michelangelo Merisi) (1571–1610) and his followers. In: *Heilbrunn Timeline of Art History*. New York, NY: The Metropolitan Museum of Art; 2000.

Langdon H. *Caravaggio: A Life*. New York, NY: Farrar, Straus and Giroux; 1999.

Martin JR. *Baroque*. New York, NY: Harper & Row; 1977.

Wheelock AK Jr. *Still Lifes of the Golden Age: Northern European Paintings from the Heinz Family Collection*. Washington, DC: The National Gallery of Art; 1989.

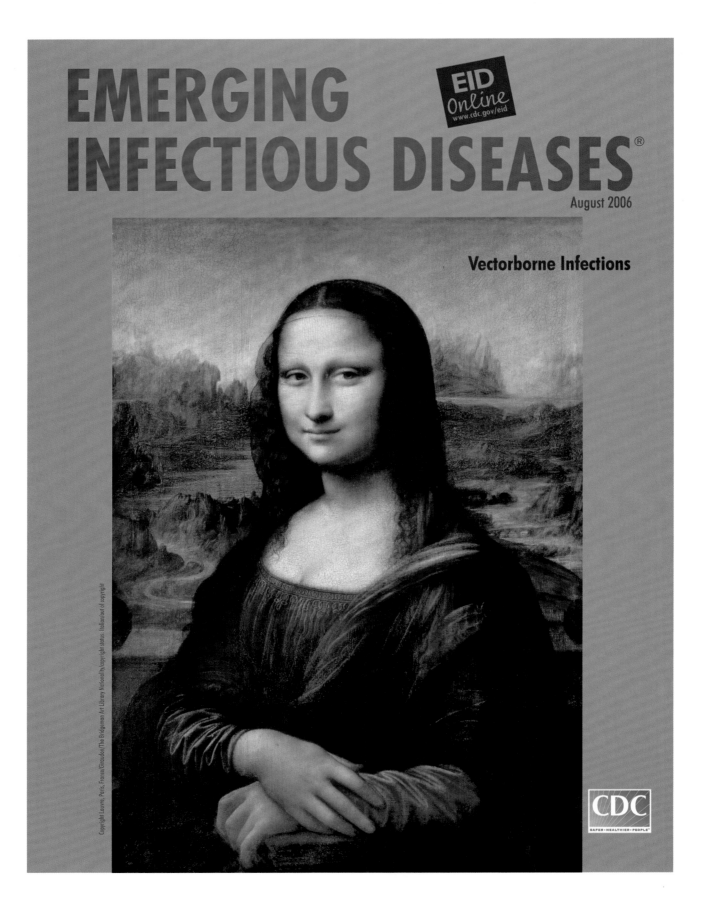

EMERGING INFECTIOUS DISEASES®

EID Online www.cdc.gov/eid

August 2006

Vectorborne Infections

Copyright Louvre, Paris, France/Giraudon/The Bridgeman Art Library Nationality/copyright status: Italian/out of copyright

CDC
SAFER·HEALTHIER·PEOPLE™

Emerg. Infect. Dis., Vol. 12, No. 8, Aug. 2006

ART, SCIENCE, AND LIFE'S ENIGMAS

Vinci, a small town near Florence, Italy, dates back to Roman times, when it was inhabited by the Etruscans. "But this town is even more renowned for having given its name to the famous Leonardo da Vinci, who, in any discipline of science and art he dedicated himself to, surpassed all his contemporaries," wrote Emanuele Repetti in his geographic dictionary of Tuscany. In the modern sense, during his lifetime, the great Leonardo had no surname—"da Vinci" means "from Vinci."

Born out of wedlock to a notary-craftsman and a peasant woman, Leonardo was nonetheless well educated in Florence. At this cultural center, home of the Medici, he was apprenticed to sculptor and painter Andrea Del Verrocchio. "Marvelous and divine, indeed, was Lionardo the son of ser Piero da Vinci," said writer and painter Giorgio Vasari in his *Lives of the Artists*. During his apprenticeship, charged with painting an angel in Verrocchio's *The Baptism of Christ*, he painted a face so divine that Verrocchio never touched colors again, "angry that a boy should know more than he."

"He is a poor pupil who does not surpass his master," Leonardo noted, when his mathematical knowledge exceeded his tutor's. Botanist, architect, civil and military engineer, town planner, hydrologist, cartographer, Leonardo anticipated, 500 years ago, the scientific discoveries of our time. "He made models of mills and presses, and machines to be worked by water, and designs for tunneling through mountains, and levers and cranes for raising great weights, so that it seemed that his brain never ceased inventing; and many of these drawings are still scattered about." Though his radical notions (aviation, military hardware, mechanical calculation) escaped his contemporaries, his genius was widely acknowledged in his lifetime. Yet, much of his work has been lost to his flamboyance. Many projects were unfinished or obscured by secrecy and cryptic records. He wrote backwards with the left hand, so notes meant for him alone could be read only in the mirror. Only a dozen or so paintings survive.

At age 30, handsome and gifted, a musician who improvised verses on a lute of his own invention, Leonardo owned a studio in Milan and had several apprentices. He completed his first large painting, *Virgin of the Rocks*, and the masterpiece *Last Supper*. Then, he went to Venice and back to Florence to work as military engineer. He traveled to Mantua and Rome, where Raphael and Michelangelo worked, then to Pavia and Bologna. Finally, he left Italy for France and the court of humanist King Francis I. Though he painted little in France, he brought with him some of his great works, including *Mona Lisa*, which remained there after his death in the king's arms at age 67.

Art and science were aligned harmoniously in Leonardo. Art was guided by science, and science was expressed through art. His studies and experiments, begun in Verrocchio's workshop, mentioned in his correspondence with Ludovico, and recorded in copious notebooks, are masterfully illustrated. To paint better, he studied anatomy, dissecting human bodies and drawing them in detail. His work with optics, especially prisms, which anticipated Newton's, refined his rendition of light and shadow. His figures showing insertion of the muscles and their movements are still admired by anatomists. "It is true that decorum should be observed," he believed, "that is, movements should announce the motion of the mind of the one who is moving."

"Lionardo was so pleased whenever he saw a strange head or beard or hair of unusual appearance that he would follow such a person a whole day, and so learn him by heart, that when he reached home he could draw him as if he were present." Guided less by his extraordinary talent and more by meticulous technique, he shunned tradition and theory. In the most ubiquitous portrait of all time, *Mona Lisa*, which graces museums, dormitories, billboards, wine bottles, and a cover of *Emerging Infectious Diseases*, the artist paid lip service to the formal vocabulary of Florentine tradition: a half-length figure, turned almost directly toward the viewer, beauty emanating from inner virtue.

Then, he positioned the figure up front to increase drama and intensity. Breaking with tradition, he painted a landscaped background, spatial depth. Instead of outlining the portrait, he merged it with surroundings. Perfecting sfumato, a technique described in antiquity by Pliny, he created an imperceptible transition between light and dark and sometimes between colors, "smoking" harsh edges with brushstrokes invisible to the naked eye. Cognizant of the way light fell on curved surfaces, he used layers of transparent color to capture it on gauzy veil or skin. The result was ethereal, magical, a glow that transformed portraiture for the ages, demanding not just likeness but the embodiment of spirit.

"As art may imitate nature, she does not appear to be painted, but truly of flesh and blood. On looking closely at the pit of her throat, one could swear that the pulses were beating," wrote Vasari. *Mona Lisa*, he continued, was painted for Florentine silk merchant Francesco del Giocondo, who commissioned it for his wife Lisa Gherandini, Mona (Madame) Lisa del Giocondo (La Gioconda), to mark the birth of their second son. Leonardo worked on the painting for several years and parted with it only at death.

"Executed in a manner well calculated to astonish all who behold her," the portrait was prominently displayed, admired, and widely reproduced. Raphael created a series of portraits with a striking resemblance, and among others, dadaist Marcel Duchamp and surrealist Salvador Dalí produced their mock interpretations. Yet "those who put the moustache on Mona Lisa," wrote contemporary artist Barnett Newman, "are not attacking it or art, but Leonardo da Vinci the man. What irritates them is that this man with half a dozen pictures has this great name in history, whereas, they, with their large oeuvre, aren't sure."

"Mona Lisa being most beautiful, he used while he was painting her, to have men to sing and play to her and buffoons to amuse her, to take away that look of melancholy which is so often seen in portraits; and in this of Lionardo's there is a peaceful smile more divine than human." Much has been speculated about the smile, about the painting, about Leonardo. While Vasari was acquainted with the Giocondo family, he did not write his anecdotal biography until more than 30 years after Leonardo's death, and competing accounts of *Mona Lisa*'s origin and identity abound. If the portrait was commissioned, why was it never delivered to its patron? Leonardo himself left scant evidence of his own opinions and ideas and only one definitive self-portrait in red chalk, a venerable face carved by time, framed by flowing hair and beard.

Some attribute the uncanny perfection of *Mona Lisa* to Leonardo's scientific observation, mathematical instinct, unparalleled skill, and the harmony of the composition. Others take different paths: "The elusive quality of Mona Lisa's smile . . . is almost entirely in low spatial frequencies, and so is seen best by your peripheral vision."

The subtle smile, reminiscent of archaic funerary statues (*kouroi, korai*), the languid eyes, the puzzling backdrop of nature, the intricate loops of the neckline, the calm hands, even the absence of visible facial hair (eyebrows and eyelashes were not the style) add to the mysterious, semi-abstract quality of the face.

The enigma of Leonardo's creation and the intrigue surrounding its origin, identity, and meaning can only be a metaphor for his own life and ideas and, by extension, ours. An archetype of the Renaissance, this man who would and could do everything must have peered inside himself for answers he had sought far afield. And just as he dissected and outlined the physical body, he sought to find and paint the spirit. Always the scientist, he knew that a portrait alone, no matter how exacting, would not do. Rejecting the flat background of tradition, he added the landscape. Part dream, part romantic reality, it provided perspective and connected the figure to the world, adding to the enigma and possibly holding the definitive interpretation.

The puzzles of our era—unknown pathogens, many of them vectorborne, emerging biological threats, ecologic disasters, antimicrobial drug resistance—can also benefit from meticulous observation, accurate recording, added perspective, and the interdisciplinary approach to knowledge. Just as with Leonardo, the art is in the science.

Bibliography

BBC. Mona Lisa smile secrets revealed. February 18, 2003. Available at: http://news.bbc.co.uk/2/hi/entertainment/2775817.stm. Accessed April 25, 2013.

Repetti, E. *Dizionario geografico fisico storico della Toscana contenente la descrizione di tutti i luoghi del granducato ducato di Lucca, Garfagnana e Lunigiana.* 5 vols. and appendix. Florence; 1833–1846.

Treasures of the World. Theft of the Mona Lisa. Available at: http://www.pbs.org/treasuresoftheworld/a_nav/mona_nav/main_monafrm.html. Accessed April 25, 2013.

Vasari G. *Lives of the Artists.* London, England: Penguin Classics; 1971.

Zöllner F, Nathan J. *Leonardo da Vinci: The Complete Paintings and Drawings.* London: Taschen; 2003.

Microbial Adaptation and Change

"There are two problems in painting," said American artist Frank Stella (b. 1936) when he was still a brash young man. "One is to find out what painting is, and the other is to find out how to make a painting." Stella's interest in the definition of painting may have reflected late 19th/early 20th-century modernist concerns. More contemporary concerns focus primarily on how to make a painting and how to use materials, methods, concepts, or traditions to create a work that may not even be called a painting. *How* a work is determines *what* it is. This modern process of painting may shed light on other aspects of life, including microbial adaptation and change, one of the factors involved in disease emergence.

At one time, art was organized by schools, later by movements. Today, these designations are difficult to apply. Painting cannot be categorized exclusively as a certain palette or style, and no consistent look or theme can be used to quantify its sum. The old labels (abstract, realist, symbolist, surrealist, expressionist, narrative) may still describe some works. But others defy all convention. They have no images, no drawing, no color, no canvas, or are not made by the artist's hand.

Atlanta artist Eric Mack (b. 1976), a man of his times, is part of the contemporary scene and its pressures to create a painting. "I'm all about shape, pattern, and repetition of form," is how Mack describes his own work. Among his techniques, collage and assemblage are suited for discovering new forms and forming new ways to connect objects retrieved from the world. His canvases contain synthetic netting, natural fibers, leaves, Japanese text, board game graphics, corporate logos, small levers and sockets, plugs, dials, and switches. These bits and pieces of objects, punctuated by a painted eyeball here, a peacock feather there, are laboriously integrated into a fluid backdrop of color applied by brush or aerosol. The effect refers to recent traditions, among them abstract expressionism, pop, and graffiti.

This type of modern painting embodies the sprawl, clutter, and flux of today's human communities. Complex composites of unlikely pieces, the works portray new forms constructed out of old and attached as never before. Organic arrangements of viable human, mechanical, and environmental parts, they have rich metaphorical potential. The solid microcosms often anchored against undulating fluid, now blotted with clumps of color, now disappearing against bare canvas, encompass all, including human and microbial interaction.

"Our relationship to infectious pathogens," wrote the late Joshua Lederberg, molecular biologist also known for his work in genetics, artificial intelligence, and space exploration, "is part of an evolutionary drama. Here we are. Here are the bugs." These ubiquitous bugs have, among other advantages, the ability to change in ways that make them dangerous. For example *E. coli* O157:H7 started out as a pathogen capable of causing mild diarrhea. Newly acquired genes transformed it into a virulent microbe that also destroys kidneys and red blood cells. Diversification in some strains of group A streptococci, common bacteria that normally do not cause disease in humans, is causing the reemergence of a severe form of invasive disease.

As we cope with the evolutionary changes of microbes within our own changing environment, we have certain advantages and disadvantages. While we continue to acquire new technology (vaccines, antimicrobial drugs, diagnostic tools) and a rising life expectancy, we are handicapped by crowding and by social, political, economic, and, therefore, hygienic stratification, which provide the opportunity for infectious agents to spread with unprecedented speed across disadvantaged human populations and, from them, to everyone else.

Collage and assemblage, which work so well in contemporary art, mirror microbial activity that can cause havoc in the global community. Like the artist's bits of objects, microbial ultrastructures can reassort, recombine, and reassemble into brand new entities. They adapt to new ecologic niches or species, produce new toxins, and bypass or suppress immune defenses to infect humans and animals. Their plasticity frustrates vaccine development, and they become resistant to even the most potent drugs.

We have used drugs, vaccines, and pesticides against pathogens for a century. But because of the evolutionary potential of microbes, the very tools used to control them can promote mutations, adaptations, and migrations that enable pathogens to proliferate or nonpathogens to start causing disease. No drug is effective against all microbes, and as a drug is used, resistant microbes often emerge from the initially susceptible population.

Some strains of pathogenic bacteria are now resistant to nearly all antimicrobial drugs. Resistance is also found in the treatment of viral, fungal, and parasitic diseases. In addition, improper use and overuse of these drugs contribute to resistance. In his 1945 Nobel Prize acceptance speech, Alexander Fleming warned to no avail, "It is not difficult to make microbes resistant to penicillin in the laboratory by exposing them to concentrations not sufficient to kill them, and the same thing has occasionally happened in the body. . . . Moral: If you use penicillin, use enough."

Cover art in this chapter address disease emergence through "collage and assemblage" practiced by microbes. *Herakles and the Stymphalian Birds* links the mythical birds on an ancient Athenian black-figured amphora with migratory birds today, which introduce new flu strains into domestic poultry and swine as they fly around the globe. These strains can amplify and mutate close to human populations and increase the risk that the virus will recombine with local human strains to form a new virus with pandemic potential. Edvard Munch's famous *Self-Portrait after the*

Spanish Flu ponders the next flu pandemic likely to be brought about by flu strains arising from such antigenic shift.

Other covers in this section provide more opportunities to discuss microbial collage and assemblage. Paolo Veronese's *Venice Receives from Juno the Doge's Hat* ponders coronavirus, an old virus, which left its wildlife reservoir to cause severe acute respiratory syndrome (SARS), a lethal disease in humans. Jacques-Louis David's *Coronation of Empress Josephine* elaborates on how antigenic variation or some other unknown cause has brought obscure coronaviruses into the spotlight. Along the same lines, Anne Adams's *Pi* touches on the infectious causes of neuropathy, among them interspecies hybrids of pathogenic yeasts that can cause meningoencephalitis.

The section's final work of art, Richard Estes's *DRUGS*, with its iconic image of the corner drugstore, brings into focus the way scientists, much like artists, try to bring order in the universe through the removal of unneeded detail. After singling out microbes that cause disease, scientists create drugs to neutralize their effects on human health. For their part, the microbes expel, modify, or exclude the drugs and become resistant to them. New drugs have to be created, which will have the same fate as the cycle of antimicrobial drug resistance continues.

Bibliography

Aziz RK, Kotb M. Rise and persistence of global M1T1 clone of *Streptococcus pyogenes*. *Emerg Infect Dis.* 2008;14:1511–1517.

Lederberg J. Emerging infections: an evolutionary perspective. *Emerg Infect Dis.* 1998;3:366–371.

Potter P. Collage and assemblage in the microbial world. *Emerg Infect Dis.* 2008. Available at: http://www.cdc.gov/EID/content/14/10/1680.htm. Accessed April 25, 2013.

Schwabsky B. *Vitamin P: New Perspectives in Painting.* Boston, MA: Phaidon Press; 2004.

Stella F. Text of a lecture at the Pratt Institute. In: *The Writings of Frank Stella.* Cologne, Germany: Verlag der Buchhandlung Walther König; 2001.

Thompson J. *How to Read a Modern Painting: Lessons from the Modern Masters.* New York, NY: Harry N. Abrams; 2006.

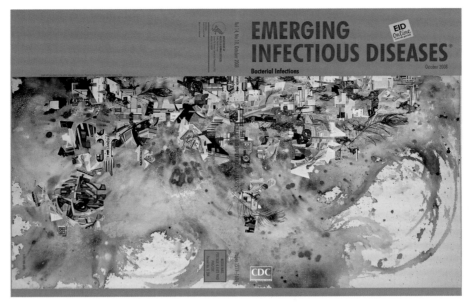

Bacterial Infections; http://dx.doi.org/10.3201/eid1410.AC1410

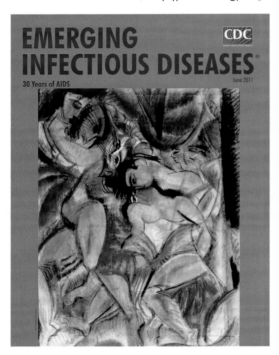

30 Years of AIDS; http://dx.doi.org/10.3201/
eid1706.AC1706

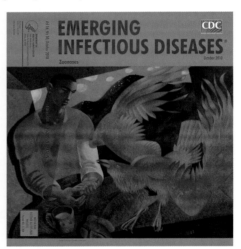

Zoonoses; http://dx.doi.org/10.3201/
eid1610.AC1610

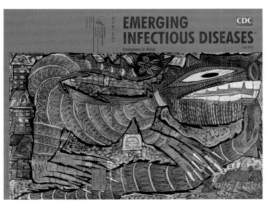

Emergence in Africa; http://dx.doi.org/10.3201/
eid1607.AC1607

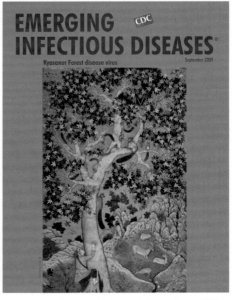

Kyasanur Forest Disease Virus; http://dx.
doi.org/10.3201/eid1509.AC1509

EMERGING
INFECTIOUS DISEASES®

August 2010

Influenza

Courtesy of Kröller-Müller Museum, Otterlo the Netherlands

NOT FROM THE STARS DO I MY JUDGMENT PLUCK[1]

"It amuses me enormously to paint the night right on the spot," wrote Vincent van Gogh to his brother Theo. "Normally, one draws and paints the painting during the daytime after the sketch. But I like to paint the thing immediately. It is true that in the darkness I can take a blue for a green, a blue lilac for a pink lilac, since it is hard to distinguish the quality of the tone. But it is the only way to get away from our conventional night with poor pale whitish light." Despite this affection for the night, van Gogh described *Night Café*, one of his best known night paintings, as "one of the ugliest I have done." Though he loved the purity of the night outdoors, he loathed urban night life. "I have attempted to show that the café is a place where a man can ruin himself, become mad, commit a crime." He moved away from Paris, where he lived with Theo, to Arles, "wishing to see a new light" and explore the calm.

In Paris he had come to know the impressionists and to experiment with broken brushstrokes and the style of the pointillists Georges Seurat and Paul Signac. He studied with Fernand Cormon and made friendships and contacts in the art world. His palette was transformed, from dark tones and stillness to yellows and blues and swirling lines. Yet, "When I left you at the station to go south," he told Theo, "I was very miserable, almost an invalid and almost a drunkard. Now at last something is beginning to show on the horizon: Hope." Moving to the countryside was an effort to get in touch with a more authentic way to live, to focus on ideas and nourish the spirituality he long sought, first as a student at the seminary and then in art.

The simplicity of rural life appealed to him on another level. "I will begin by telling you that this country seems to me as beautiful as Japan as far as the limpidity of the atmosphere and the gay color effects are concerned." Like many of his contemporaries, van Gogh was fascinated with art from the Orient. He collected and copied woodblock prints and welcomed Utagawa Hiroshige and Katsushika Hokusai into the Western vernacular. "My whole work . . . builds so to speak on what the Japanese have done." Under their influence, he moved toward color and away from naturalism, volume and perspective, light and shadow. "I envy the Japanese artists for the incredible neat clarity which all their works have. It is never boring and you never get the impression that they work in a hurry. It is as simple as breathing; they draw a figure with a couple of strokes . . . as if it were as easy as buttoning one's waistcoat."

Van Gogh's meteoric rise to greatness in the so-brief span of his 37 years took place in various settings and was marked by emotional turmoil, from unrequited love and failure at evangelism to familial strife and poverty. Through it all, he assessed his own legacy as "of very secondary importance." Largely self-taught, he absorbed brief but potent influences. He took his first artistic steps in his native Holland, copying from art books, working as apprentice for an art dealer at age 16. He received formal instruction from leading Hague School artist Anton Mauve, then moved to London, where he taught school for a couple of years. He became interested in the Barbizon group, particularly Jean-François Millet, and started to

---

1 William Shakespeare, "Sonnet 14."

paint peasants and rural life, a practice he would continue throughout his life. He traveled to Belgium to study at the Antwerp Academy, an unsuccessful venture, and soon after went to live with Theo in Paris. He took up painting in earnest in 1880 and continued until his death, producing in 10 years 900 paintings and more than 1,100 works on paper. Some of his masterpieces were created during the past 2 years of life when, overcome by mental illness, he committed himself to the asylum in Saint-Rémy. "I put my heart and my soul into my work and have lost my mind in the process."

The evening and night, recurring themes in van Gogh's work, interested him even before he began to paint. As a youth he was an avid reader, fluent in Dutch, German, English, and French. Many of the books he mentioned in his letters described the spiritual and poetic character of the night, the interval between sunset and dark, and the darkness between dusk and dawn. "It seems to me that the night is more alive and richly colored than the day." This time for reflection and introspection sparked his artistic imagination and produced, among other major works, *The Starry Night*; *Landscapes at Twilight*; *Peasant Life at Evening*; *Poetry of the Night*; and *Terrace of a Café at Night*, a painting reminiscent of Hiroshige's *Scene of the Saruwaka-cho Theater Street by Night*.

"On the terrace there are small figures of people drinking," van Gogh wrote to his brother about his first starry painting of an outdoor café. "An immense yellow lantern illuminates the terrace, the facade, the sidewalk, and even casts light on the paving stones of the road, which take a pinkish violet tone. The gables of the houses, like a fading road below a blue sky studded with stars, are dark blue or violet with a green tree." Excited about the results, he explained to Theo, "Here you have a night painting without black, with nothing but beautiful blue and violet and green and in this surrounding the illuminated area colors itself sulfur pale yellow and citron green."

In this and other night paintings, he struggled to achieve luminosity with contrasting or exaggerated colors and to demonstrate the superiority of natural light and the imagination over artificial light and reality. He struggled equally to express the mysterious influence of the night on the human heart as he understood it from his own tumultuous life. "I am a man of passion, capable and prone to undertake more or less foolish things which I happen to repent more or less." While he worked on his first painting of a starry night, he wrote, "It is good for me to work hard. But that does not keep me from having a terrible need of—shall I say the word—yes, of religion. Then I go out at night to paint the stars."

This need went back to van Gogh's days as evangelist in an impoverished mining town in Belgium. He was dismissed from that post for showing extreme charity and identifying too much with the flock. His religious zeal dampened, he vowed then to make art for the common people, to paint them and their concerns. And who among the common people has not gazed upward wishing to decipher the mysteries of the sky? "Looking at the stars always makes me dream," he wrote, "Why, I ask myself, shouldn't the shining dots of the sky be as accessible as the black dots on the map of France?" Like others throughout the ages, he sought solace in the stars' mysterious light and viewed them as symbols of hope. "Just as we take the train to get to Tarascon or Rouen, we take death to reach a star."

The stars, and their influence on human life—domain of the scientist, let alone the lover and the poet—have roots in antiquity and were examined long before van Gogh swirled them down to earth for all to see. In the 14th century, Italian physicians ascribed a mysterious illness often turned epidemic to the adverse influence of the stars and called it *influentia*. The term *influenza* was first used in English in 1743 during an outbreak of the disease in Europe. Despite our continued inability to prevent its global spread, we have learned since that viruses are the culprits and that influenza has less to do with ethereal substances emanating from the stars and more with tiny droplets shared generously between patrons under the café awning and in other gathering places. We are still just as intrigued with the stars and van Gogh's interpretations. And we have astronomy, as the Bard put it, "But not to tell of good or evil luck, / Of plagues, of dearths, or seasons' quality."

Bibliography

Blumer D. The illness of Vincent van Gogh. *Am J Psychiatry*. 2002;159:519–526.

The Complete Letters of Vincent van Gogh. Boston, MA: Bullfinch Press of Little Brown and Co; 2000.

Druick DW, Kort ZP. *Van Gogh and Gauguin: The Studio of the South*. New York, NY: Thames and Hudson; 2002.

Gift TL, Palekar RS, Sodha SV, et al. Household effects of school closure during pandemic (H1N1) 2009, Pennsylvania, USA. *Emerg Infect Dis*. 2010;16:1315–1317.

Kendall R. *Van Gogh's van Goghs: Masterpieces from the van Gogh Museum, Amsterdam*. Washington, DC: National Gallery of Art; 1998.

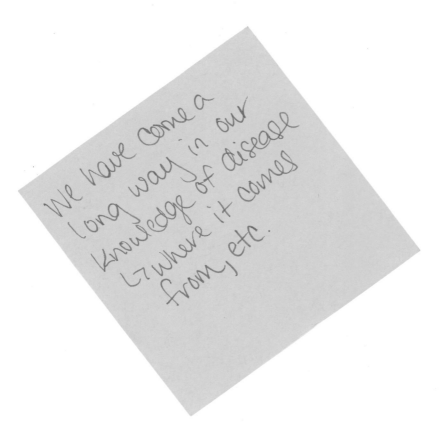

We have come a long way in our knowledge of disease ⌐7 where it comes from, etc.

EMERGING
INFECTIOUS DISEASES

EID Online
www.cdc.gov/eid

A Peer-Reviewed Journal Tracking and Analyzing Disease Trends

Vol.11, No.8, August 2005

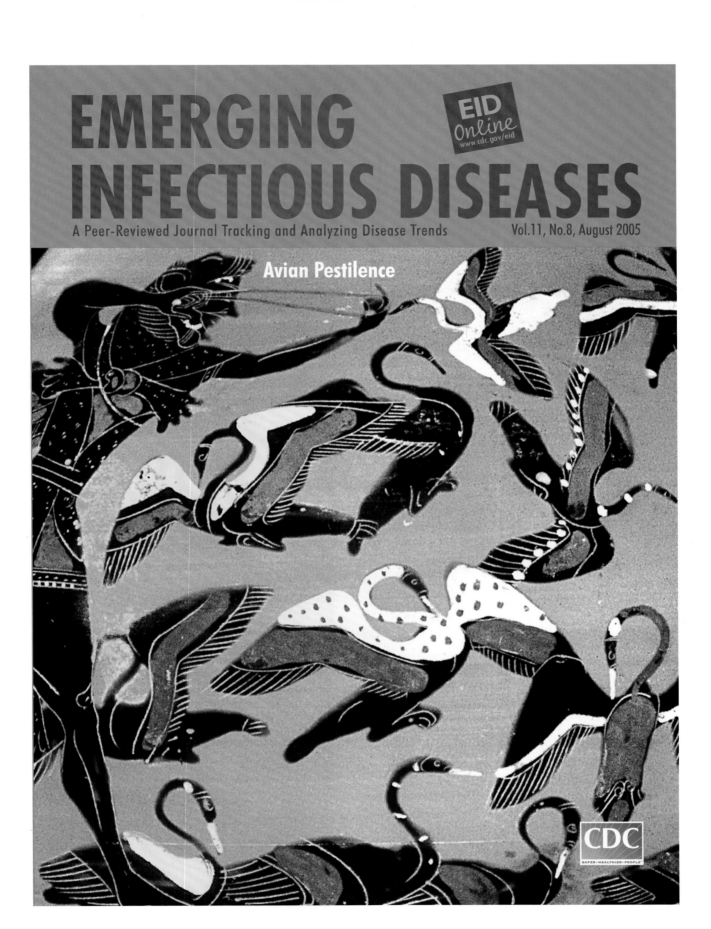

Avian Pestilence

CDC
SAFER·HEALTHIER·PEOPLE™

ANCIENT MYTHS AND AVIAN PESTILENCE

"These birds are the size of a crane and are like the ibis, but their beaks are more powerful, and not crooked like the ibis," wrote ancient traveler and writer, Pausanias. He was referring to large flocks of metal-clawed ornithes, which according to legend, roosted in the dense marshes around Lake Stymphalis in Arcadia, ravaging crops and the livelihood of neighboring villages. This scourge, he speculated, was not local. "The Arabian Desert breeds, among other wild creatures, birds . . . which are quite as savage against men as lions or leopards. . . . These fly against those who come to hunt them, wounding and killing them with their beaks."

The flesh-eating predators further terrorized local inhabitants by dispatching against them razor-edged feathers like arrows. "All armor of bronze or iron that men wear is pierced by the birds," elaborated Pausanias. Pets of Ares, god of war, these birds were a public menace too great for the community to control, a challenge finally assigned, along with other "labors," to strongman of all time, Herakles.

Son of Zeus and mortal Alcmene, Herakles might have enjoyed the privileged life of a demigod. But, victimized by Zeus's jealous wife, Hera, he endured a mortal lot of labor and hardship, punctuated by periods of madness and aberrant behavior. Strong, resourceful, and gifted with magical defenses, he had to struggle, nonetheless, against nature that was deadly, unpredictable, and arbitrary. During his celebrated labors, he battled vicious beasts (among them Kerberos, the guard of Hades) and cleaned out the infamous Augean Stables, which housed the filthiest herd of cattle in Hellas. To attain immortality, he performed, as penance for his misdeeds, arduous service to the community, using his unparalleled strength to support his fellow humans.

The thick marsh habitat of the Stymphalian birds worked against Herakles. His bow and arrows failed, for he could neither see nor reach the birds through the dense vegetation. Only asked to drive them away, he abandoned efforts to eliminate the birds; instead, he conned them into leaving the area on their own. With a pair of krotala (metal rattles) made by Hephaestus, god of the forge, Herakles frightened the birds out of their refuge and chased them as they flew east to the Isle of Ares in the Black Sea.

Herakles and the Stymphalian Birds adorns a black-figured amphora, a ceramic vase popular in ancient Athens. Such vases were made of iron-rich clay and decorated with black silhouettes in mythical heroic scenes. Illustrations were incised and painted with a slip (liquid clay), which turned black during firing without oxygen.

The scene is full of action but contains no background clues. Hellenic myths focus on the here and now and its terrifying uncertainties and dilemmas. They address human concerns, not philosophical conceit. Their narrative blurs the boundaries of history and legend as heroes cross back and forth from fantasy to reality, often operating in geographic locations that can never quite be verified on a map.

Herakles cuts a powerful figure as he leans forward, aiming a sling at the birds. His body, draped with the impenetrable hide of the Nemean Lion, a trophy from his first labor, forms a barrier against the flock. The birds scatter in disarray, not laden with metal as the myth prescribes, but confused, half resting at the foot of the hero, half flapping their wings against each other, compromised by the lack of cover. These are beautiful birds, dotted and striped, with elegant long necks turned defensively inward. Yet, in some versions of the Stymphalian labor, the birds are harpies—half metal-feathered ornithes, half human heads with bronze beaks.

Herakles probably wished he had not stopped at chasing these Arabian birds away from Arcadia for, even in the small world of antiquity, geographic migration ruled. The birds surfaced again, during his sail with Jason and the Argonauts in search of the Golden Fleece, to be chased away again, this time by the sons of the North Wind.

Flawed humanity tested by overwhelming challenges rings true today. Heroic figures battling great odds excite our collective imagination. And public challenges (waste pollution out of control, avian pestilence) have changed little. Waterfowl, a benign species, were demonized in the Stymphalian myth, their hideous mien likely borne of human fear and helplessness, for who knows what pestilence they had inflicted on the community around the lake. And each time those birds flew to a new place, they had contact with other birds and opportunities for genetic reassortment, redistribution, and modification of pathogens throughout the migratory route.

Resistant to slings and arrows and prone to long-distance migrations, birds such as the ones on this amphora persist beyond our ancestors' morbid imaginations. Not because of mythical metal paraphernalia but for their explosive potential as natural reservoirs and amplifying hosts of pathogens. Viremic migratory birds acting as introductory hosts may have brought West Nile virus to the Western Hemisphere, perhaps by infecting ornithophilic mosquitoes, which may have infected amplifying hosts and eventually humans.

Migratory waterfowl (ducks, geese) also carry flu viruses in their intestines and shed them in their secretions and excretions. As these waterfowl migrate around the globe, they introduce new flu strains into domestic poultry and swine. These strains can then amplify and mutate close to human populations, increasing the risk that the virus will recombine with local human strains to form a new virus with pandemic potential. Like the legendary harpies, these new strains, half human half avian, pose an immense public health challenge.

We now know more about bird pestilence. West Nile virus infection and avian flu are just as ominous as razor-edged feathers. And while Herakles had krotala from the gods, we must work with human tools: repellants and pesticides, vaccines, antiviral drugs, or medical isolation and quarantine.

Bibliography

Daum LT, Shaw MW, Klimov AI, et al. Influenza A (H3N2) outbreak, Nepal. *Emerg Infect Dis.* 2005;11:1186–1191.

Hayes EB, Komar N, Nasci RS, et al. Epidemiology and dynamics of transmission of West Nile virus disease. *Emerg Infect Dis.* 2005;11:1167–1179.

Metropolitan Museum of Art. Athenian vase painting: red-and black-figure techniques. Available at: http://www.metmuseum.org/toah/hd/vase/hd_vase.htm. Accessed April 24, 2013.

Mills A. *Mythology: Myths, Legends, and Fantasies.* Hong Kong: Global Book Publishing; 2004.

Pausanias. *Pausanias: Description of Greece: Attica and Corinth; Books I-II.* Cambridge, MA: Harvard University Press; 1918.

Rappole JH, Derrickson SR, Hubálek Z. Migratory birds and spread of West Nile virus in the Western Hemisphere. *Emerg Infect Dis.* 2000;6:319–328.

EMERGING
INFECTIOUS DISEASES

EID Online www.cdc.gov/eid

A Peer-Reviewed Journal Tracking and Analyzing Disease Trends   Vol.9, No.3, March 2003

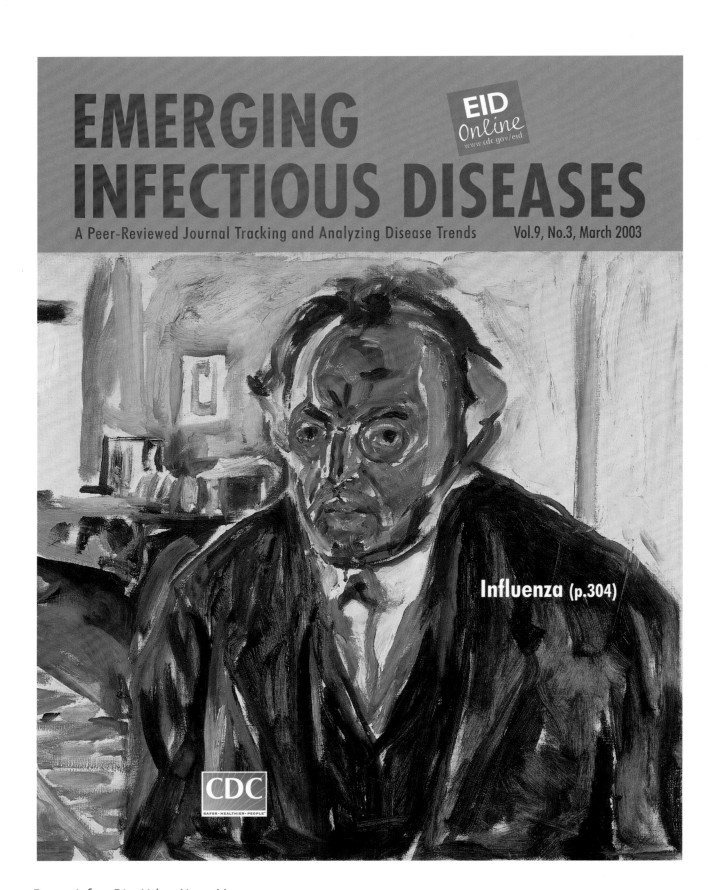

Influenza (p.304)

CDC
SAFER·HEALTHIER·PEOPLE™

THE HUMAN FACE OF PESTILENCE

"Illness, insanity, and death . . . kept watch over my cradle and accompanied me all my life," noted innovative Norwegian artist Edvard Munch. Deeply affected by the untimely death of his mother when he was 5 and his 15-year-old sister when he was 14, he devoted his early artistic efforts to painting their predicament and the ravages of tuberculosis, "the wan face in profile against the pillow, the despairing mother at the bedside, the muted light, the tousled hair, the useless glass of water."

His own fragile physical and emotional state dominated the way he viewed and executed his art. In his middle years, incapacitated by depression, he spent time in a sanatorium in Denmark, and even though he recovered, his work never regained its initial expressiveness.

Munch studied in Oslo and traveled extensively to Italy, Germany, and France, where he took in the influences of his contemporaries (Toulouse-Lautrec, van Gogh, Gauguin), who were turning the angst of modern civilization into symbolism and stark expressionism. Preoccupation with decadence and evil pervaded the artistic and literary climate of the day. Darkness and horror inspired deeply personal, highly expressive art in a variety of styles, all of which fit under the umbrella of symbolism, as long as they embodied its peculiarly gloomy state of mind. The movement's emphasis on inner vision rather than observation of nature captured Munch's haunted imagination and engaged his moody genius.

Inspired by the work of Henrik Ibsen, Munch studied psychoanalysis and created art that unraveled the mysteries of the psyche. His canvases are filled with agonizing uncertainty and excruciating loneliness, anticipating Ingmar Bergman's theater and cinematic work. His personal neuroses and physical ailments permeate the cultural anxiety expressed in his work.

Even as he painted the existential drama of his own life, Munch did so without graphic depictions of monsters or apparitions. Rather, he provoked emotional response through unnatural color, internal rhythm, and undulating lines, as in *The Scream*, one of the most reproduced and universally acclaimed paintings in the history of art. Munch's ambitious (unfinished) work, *The Frieze of Life*, comprised a sequence of connected panels intended to expose the illusory nature of optimism and bring to public view the painter's innermost feelings about life—from birth to death.

Pestilence, which traumatized Munch's early years in the form of tuberculosis, continued to rule his life. In *Self-Portrait after the Spanish Flu*, the tormented painter appears judge and victim of this pandemic killer. The terse yet unsteady demeanor, the puffy discolored glare, the quivering lines of fever and chills, only highlight the despair and isolation of the "grippe" patient, the oppression, the weakness, the malaise, the lack of air, the stupor, the hopelessness.

Munch's preoccupation with suffering in this self-portrait is fully understood by those who study the Spanish flu pandemic. Erupting during the final stages of World War I, this global disaster reinforced the era's nihilism and apocalyptic visions of despair. "I had a little bird / Its name was Enza / I opened the window / And in-flew-enza," morbidly sang the children as they skipped rope. Specimens from the remains of flu victims buried in permafrost provide some clues about the

1918–19 strain. Highly contagious and unusually virulent, the deadly flu circled the globe, taking its toll among the youngest and healthiest. Medicine was then only beginning to understand infectious diseases and to take modest steps toward diagnostics and therapy.

Infectious disease medicine has come a long way, yet Munch's specter of the flu is alarmingly current. Surveillance of circulating viruses is increasing and flu vaccination has entered the mainstream, but epidemics are still frequent and strains arising from antigenic shift keep the next flu pandemic just around the corner.

Bibliography

Crawford R. The Spanish Flu. In: *Stranger than Fiction: Vignettes of San Diego History*. San Diego, CA: San Diego Historical Society; 1995.

Gibson M. *Symbolism*. New York, NY: Taschen America; 1997.

EMERGING
INFECTIOUS DISEASES®

September 2007

Coronaviruses

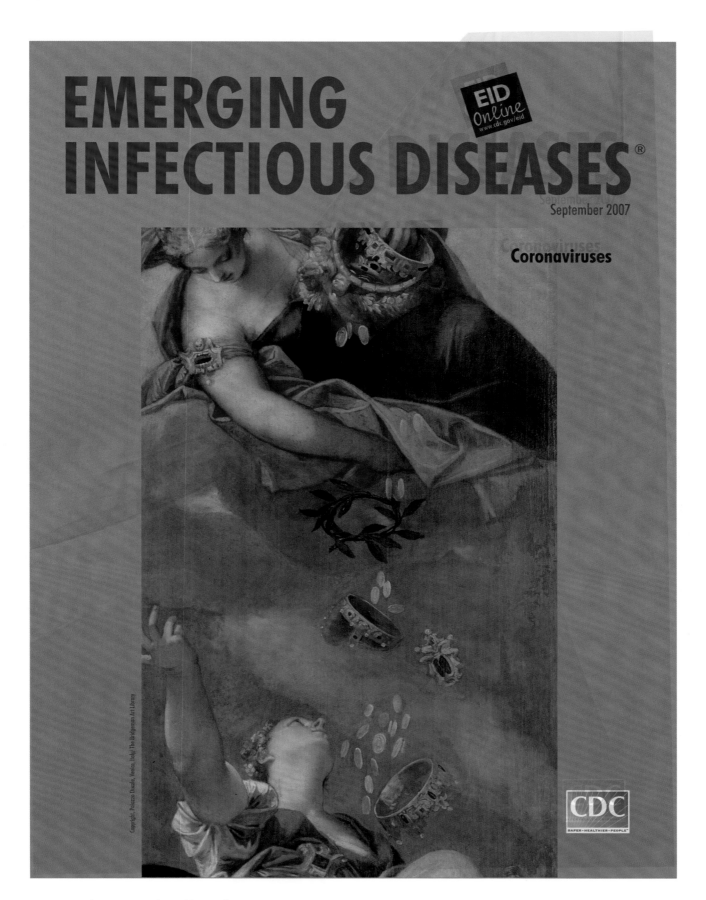

Copyright: Palazzo Ducale, Venice, Italy/The Bridgeman Art Library

NATURE HATH FRAM'D STRANGE FELLOWS IN HER TIME[2]

Painters take the same license as poets and madmen, Paolo Veronese told the Inquisition Tribunal in Venice during an interrogation. Buffoons, drunkards, exotic creatures, and anachronisms in his *Last Supper* were placed there "so they might be of service because it seemed to me fitting" in creating the scene, not as irreverence. The dispute was resolved by changing the name of the painting to *Supper in the House of Levi*. Veronese was not interested in piety or historical accuracy. Large banquets were opportunities to create feasts for the eyes, monumental gatherings framed in architectural detail, bathed in sumptuous color.

The son of a stone mason known only as Gabriele, the painter adopted the name Caliari and later became known as Veronese from his birthplace. A precocious child entirely uninterested in stone cutting, he was quickly recognized for facility with the brush and was trained by local masters Antonio Badile and Giovanni Caroto. Then, according to chronicler Giorgio Vasari, architect and engineer Michele Sanmicheli took him under his wing and "treated him like a son." He painted his first works in Verona and Mantua, but when called to Venice on a commission, he remained there for the rest of his life, becoming a preeminent master of the late Renaissance, along with Titian and Tintoretto. In the Doge's palace, the Church of San Sebastiano, the Villa Barbaro at Maser with the great architect Andrea Palladio, and churches and palaces all over the city, he extolled youth, beauty, and prodigious harvests in frescoes and oil paintings of enduring charm. A kind and amiable man, Veronese was well liked and appreciated, one of the first painters whose work was sought by collectors during his lifetime.

Early training in the mannerist style, which emphasized the decorative, was transformed by the styles of Venice, an innate sense of composition, and his genius as draftsman. He reveled in rich textures and patterns and captured luminescence in flesh and fabric, lace or wool. He was "the greatest colorist who ever lived," wrote French critic Théophile Gautier, "greater than Titian, Rubens, or Rembrandt" because he created light without violent contrasts and maintained the strength of hue and shadow, which French master Eugène Delacroix (1798–1863) said, "We are always told is impossible."

An expert illusionist, Veronese overcame the problems of applying linear perspective to the concave surfaces of church domes, overriding the architecture, simulating limitless space. With *sotto in su* techniques, he created foreshortened figures to be seen from below as floating above the viewer. He moved adventurously between secular and religious themes, incorporated classical and mythologic figures, crafted allegorical pageants, mingled the sacred with what some thought the profane.

Venice, la Serenissima or Most Serene Republic, and the myths surrounding her mercantile empire lent themselves to the theatrical, apotheotic exuberance of Veronese's style. The city, described by Petrarch in 1364 as "rich in gold but richer

---

2 William Shakespeare, *The Merchant of Venice*.

in renown," mythologized herself—Venetia, Queen of the Andriatic, at once pagan and medieval, her heritage not so much of classical Rome but the Byzantine East. He painted her effortless grandeur in gowns of gold brocade, seated on clouds, trumpeted by angels, showered with jewels from the gods.

Venice inspired generations of poets and writers from William Shakespeare and Lord Byron to Thomas Mann. And Veronese influenced the course of European art—in the 17th century through Rubens and Velazquez, in the 18th, through Giovanni Battista Tiepolo and others.

Juno, the Roman goddess bestowing gifts on Venice in Veronese's brilliant allegory *Venice Receives from Juno the Doge's Hat*, was none other than Greek goddess Hera, powerful wife of Zeus. In antiquity, her giving was legend, for havoc as well as gifts. She ruined foes but sanctioned marriage, her generosity even celebrated by Shakespeare, "Honour, riches, marriage-blessing, / Long continuance, and increasing, / Hourly joys be still upon you! / Juno sings her blessings on you." In this, another of her less bellicose appearances, Juno rains gold and crowns on Venice, grooming her for greatness and prosperity. Afloat in sensuous color, she glances down at her. An olive branch, signifying honor, acknowledges a city "mighty in her resources but mightier in virtue."

The extravagance of Juno's gesture and its gracious acceptance bespeak the mythic greatness and splendor of Venice. Poetry and utopian texts, as well as the art of Veronese's time, attributed this greatness in part to topography—though lapped by the waves, Venice maintained close ties with the northern mainland and amassed a land empire, the *terraferma* (dry land). Another link to greatness was harmonious interaction with nature and the cosmos. Venetian humanist Pietro Bembo proposed "ideal love" as key to this interaction. Likewise, Jacopo Sannazzaro in L'Arcadia (1500) attributed moral and spiritual perfection to human connection with the natural world and its rhythms.

La Serenissima succumbed in the late 1700s, becoming a *ville crépusculaire* (city like any other). Like the original Arcadia, she had existed largely in the imagination. Connection with nature, indispensable to the myth, survived the fall of the empire; poets, painters, and scientists still seek it in Venice and elsewhere.

Bejeweled crowns from above, royal coronas, seem far removed from nature. Yet nature disperses her own, less conspicuously but with far more bountiful abundance than Juno. Coronaviruses, common viruses of animals and humans, are named for their crownlike appearance. Recently, they came under the spotlight, when an obscure animal coronavirus left its wildlife reservoir to cause SARS, a lethal disease in humans. Nature's gift that keeps on giving, these viruses continue to emerge, in more species, more places, and now perhaps in North American bats, which could become involved in future emergence in humans or other animals.

Bibliography

Dominguez SR, O'Shea TJ, Oko LM, et al. Detection of group 1 coronaviruses in bats in North America. *Emerg Infect Dis.* 2007;13:1295–1300.

Dunkerton J, Foister S, Penny N. *Dürer to Veronese: Sixteenth-Century Painting in the National Gallery.* London, England: National Gallery Publications; 1999.

Eisler C. *Masterworks in Berlin: A City's Paintings Reunited*. Boston, MA: Little Brown; 1996.

Rearick WR. *The Art of Paolo Veronese 1528–1588*. Washington, DC: National Gallery of Art; 1988.

Rosand D, ed. *Titian: His World and His Legacy*. New York, NY: Columbia University Press; 1982.

Shakespeare W. *The Tempest*; Act VI, Scene 1. 1822-25. http://www.opensourceshakespeare. org/views/plays/play_view.php?WorkID=tempest&Act=4&Scene=1&Scope=scene; accessed June 11, 2013.

Vasari G. *Lives of the Artists*. London, England: Penguin Classics; 1971.

Virtus Romana and the myth of Venice. Available at: http://rubens.anu.edu.au/; accessed July 18, 2007.

EMERGING
INFECTIOUS DISEASES

EID Online
www.cdc.gov/eid

A Peer-Reviewed Journal Tracking and Analyzing Disease Trends   Vol.9, No.10, October 2003

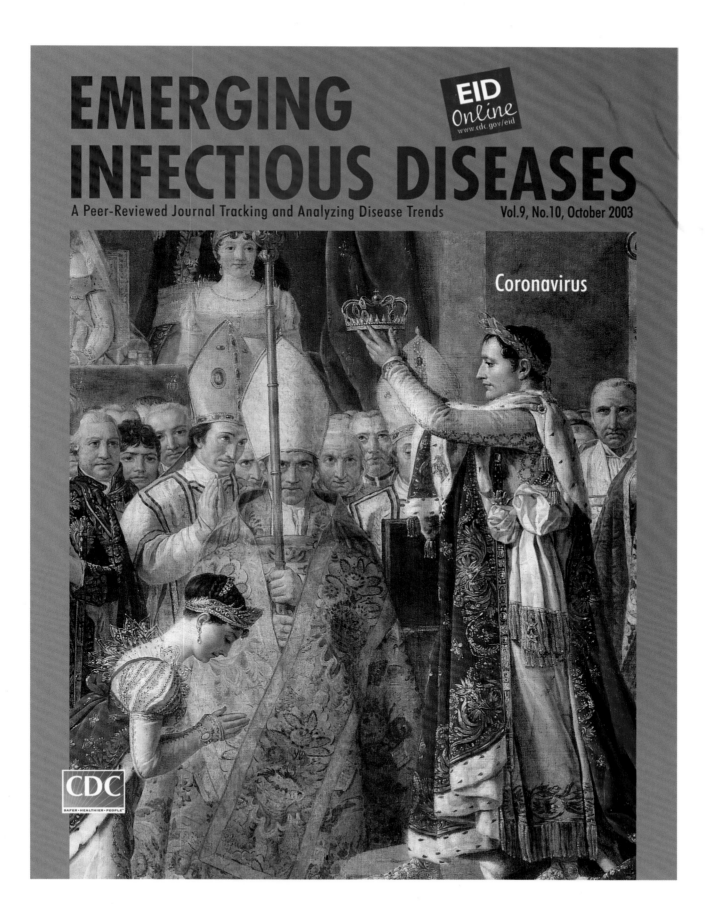

Coronavirus

CDC
SAFER·HEALTHIER·PEOPLE

CORONA OF POWER OR HALO OF DISASTER

"I was always hiding behind the instructor's chair, drawing for the duration of the class," admitted Jacques-Louis David, acknowledging his early artistic bent. The orphaned son of a wealthy Paris family, David went on to study art, first under distant relative François Boucher, then under gifted teacher and rococo painter Joseph-Marie Vien. Later, in Italy for 5 years, David became engrossed in archaeology, classical architecture, and mythology, which, along with the paintings of his compatriot Nicolas Poussin, provided inspiration for his work as leading neoclassical painter.

David's era was the Age of Enlightenment, whose standard-bearers (David Hume, Voltaire, Jean-Jacques Rousseau, Heinrich Heine) revolutionized economics, politics, and religion, steering them away from authoritarian tradition, toward reason and the common good. The arts, abandoning the baroque, relinquished the ornate, aristocratic, and frivolous excesses of rococo. They turned toward nature and heroic morality, and by extension, toward the ancient "apostles of reason," the classics, and their "noble simplicity and calm grandeur." Italy's artistic leadership declined, leaving the role of guardian of Western art to France and the students of Vien.

The great political upheavals of the mid-18th century, the American Revolution and the French Revolution, followed the sweeping changes in the world of ideas and ushered in the modern era. David enthusiastically took part in the French Revolution and interpreted the issues of his day in masterpieces drawn from ancient moral dilemmas (*The Death of Socrates*) and contemporary events (*The Death of Marat*).

Napoleon Bonaparte rose to power after a coup d'état in 1799. A plebiscite in 1802 confirmed his lifetime rule as Consul of France, in preparation for his becoming Emperor of the French Republic. In 1804, in an elaborate ceremony reminiscent of the coronation of Holy Roman Emperor Charlemagne and in the presence of Pope Pius VII, Napoleon grasped his sword to his heart and put the crown on his own head. David, then official painter to the emperor, was tasked with commemorating the coronation festivities at the cathedral of Notre Dame. David's rendition of the event does not dwell on Napoleon's imperial indiscretion. Rather, it portrays the crowning, by the emperor, of his wife, Josephine. Josephine's coronation itself is a small part of the massive composition, an enormous group portrait of more than 100 figures.

Art has been a powerful instrument of revolutions, and David used it often to portray Napoleon as legendary opponent of absolutism, embodying the quest for truth and liberty. Music has similarly served popular uprisings. Beethoven's Third Symphony, Eroica, for a brief time referred to as the Bonaparte Symphony, was inspired by Napoleon's heroic promise. This epic symphony, which dramatically captures the spirit of humanity, parallels the complexity of revolutionary passions.

In the eyes of the world, as in the eyes of those attending the lavish coronation in David's painting, Napoleon's fall came the moment he assumed imperial status. The laurel leaf crown of Roman emperors was no simple corona. To the champions of equality it symbolized tyranny. David's political entanglement with the Napoleonic era ended in imprisonment and exile. The dedication to Napoleon in Beethoven's score of the Eroica was retracted. And Josephine was banished to make room for Napoleon's true mistress, power.

The crown and its elusive promise have downed many a revolutionary hero, the corona of power often becoming halo of disaster. The same is true at times in nature. Some biologic agents are reminiscent of the sun, whose corona is only visible during a full eclipse. The coronaviruses, named for their crownlike appearance in which a loosely wound center is neatly surrounded by club-shaped peplomers, are a case in point. Known animal pathogens for many years, the more than 15 species of coronaviruses infected a variety of mammals and birds yet remained largely obscure, until antigenic variation or some other, unknown cause brought them into the spotlight. An animal pathogen causing zoonotic infection in humans or a recombinant of human coronavirus and animal virus, SARS virus has brought on a halo of disaster, circling the globe with illness and death.

Bibliography

Brinton WM. An abridged history of Europe; http://www.European-history.com/davidJl.html; accessed July 15, 2003

Glesner ES. Ludwig van Beethoven—Symphony no.3, op.55 "Eroica;" http://w3.rz-berlin.mpg.de/cmp/Beethoven_sym3.html; accessed July 15, 2003

Louvre Museum Official Website-Paintings / text. Louis David [cited 2003 Jul]. http://www.louvre.fr/anglais/collec/peint/inv3699/txt3699.htm; accessed July 15, 2003.

Vess D. The French Revolution; http://www.faculty.de.gcsu.edu/~dvess/ids/fap/frenchrev.htm; accessed July 15, 2003.

EMERGING INFECTIOUS DISEASES®

EID Online
www.cdc.gov/eid

July 2008

Central Nervous System

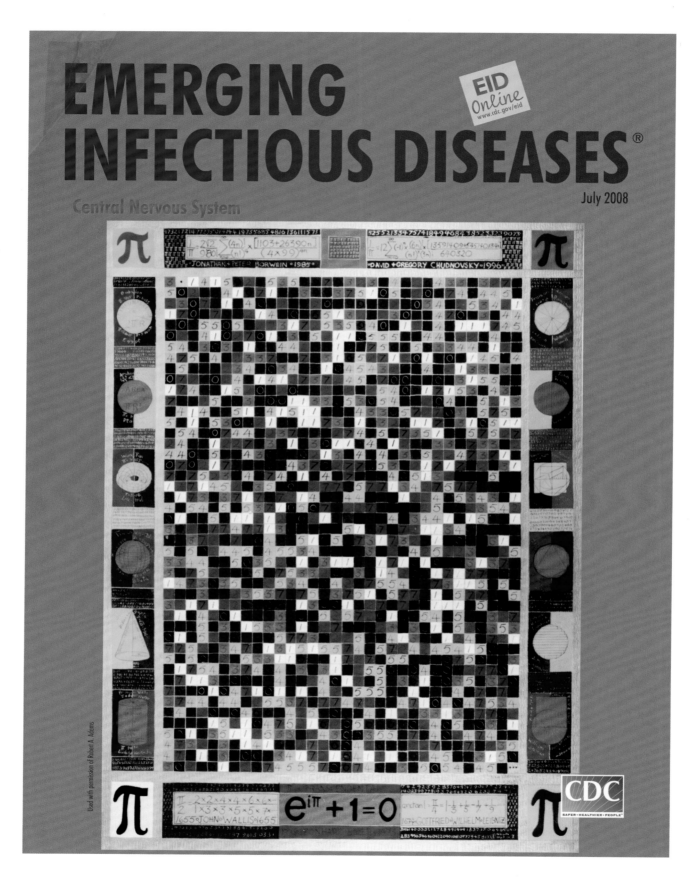

Used with permission of Robert A. Adams

MUCH MADNESS IS DIVINEST SENSE[3]

"And yet I still had so much music in my head," lamented Maurice Ravel (1875–1937) near the end of his life. The French composer was frustrated by symptoms of an undiagnosed neurologic disorder that interfered with his ability to move, speak, or express creative ideas. Now labeled primary progressive aphasia-related illness, the disorder also marked the life and art of Anne Adams.

A native of Canada, Adams was educated in the sciences and excelled in physics and chemistry, which she taught at the college level. During an interval from academe, she raised her four children, then returned to the sciences at age 35 as a student of cell biology, professor, and researcher. At age 46, she left again, this time to nurse her son, who had been injured in an automobile wreck. The injury resolved much faster than anyone expected, but Adams decided not to return to science but pursue other interests. A lover of music and the arts, she had dabbled with painting in her earlier years, mostly architectural drawing and watercolor in a classical style.

Over the next few years, she became increasingly absorbed with art, devoting all her days to work in her studio. Her style and technique evolved rapidly, and she started experimenting, particularly with expression of sounds as visual forms. She interpreted musical scores and converted them to colorful images (Rondo alla Turquoise, Rhapsody in Blue). She became fascinated with the music of Maurice Ravel, particularly his one-movement orchestral piece Boléro.

"Don't you think this theme has an insistent quality?" Ravel asked his friend Gustave Samazeuilh as he fingered the initial melody on the piano. "I'm going to try and repeat it a number of times without any development, gradually increasing the orchestra as best I can." This he did. Two melodic themes were repeated eight times over 340 bars. Volume and instrumentation increased along with two alternating staccato bass lines. There was no key change until the 326th bar, when the piece accelerated into a collapsing finale. The result was haunting and infectious, an exercise in compulsion, some said perseveration.

Ravel wrote this his best-known composition while on vacation in the south of France. He was 53. Though the musical scores were marred with spelling errors, he was not yet incapacitated by illness. The success of Boléro, which he had assessed as "a piece for orchestra without music," surprised him. During the premier of the work, a woman was said to exclaim that the composer was mad. Ravel later remarked that she must have understood the piece.

Anne Adams knew nothing of Ravel's illness or her own. But at age 53, she started to work on the painting *Unraveling Boléro*, a visual analysis of Ravel's composition. She transformed the music into colorful figures, one for each bar. Highly structured and rendered with meticulous detail, they resembled spiky space-age lace hung out to dry in neat monotonous rows. The height of figures corresponded with volume, the shape with note quality, the color with pitch.

In *Pi*, painted when Adams was 58 and before any symptoms of language loss, she moved away from translating music toward abstraction. At the peak of her creativity, she painted mathematical concepts. And it is not surprising that she chose to paint π,

---

3 Emily Dickinson, "Much Madness is divinest Sense."

one of the most mysterious and recognizable numbers, even to those who have long forgotten what it represents or how frequently it turns up in science and nature. Inside an iconic border summarizing the history of π, Adams portrayed a 32- × 46-digit portion in a matrix of the first 1,471 digits (plus the decimal point). With white, black, and component colors of the white light spectrum marking each integer from 0 to 9, she tried to capture the randomness of π's expansion.

Loss of language (difficulty with grammar, syntax, articulation, speech) and motor function (declining muscle control), main symptoms of Adams's (and Ravel's) illness, have long been known to neurologists as the result of lesions on the left frontal lobe. What was extraordinary in these two cases was the simultaneous increase in capabilities of the posterior right region of the brain. Ravel died at 62 of complications after neurosurgical treatment, Adams at 67 of aspiration pneumonia brought on by severe motor and respiratory decline.

Neuropathy, with its dreaded sequelae, is a common prospect for an aging population, and not only as it relates to primary progressive aphasia. Meningitis, the scourge of children and youth as well as the immunocompromised, has multiple infectious causes and disastrous outcomes when left undiagnosed and untreated. The epidemiology of bacterial meningitis around the world keeps evolving, impeding vaccine development. Illness caused by emerging pathogens (e.g., *Rickettsia felis*) is likely underreported. Meanwhile interspecies hybrids of pathogenic yeasts that can cause meningoencephalitis (e.g., *Cryptococcus neoformans* and *C. gattii*) are now found in patients with weakened immune systems.

Unlike Adams and Ravel, most patients with neurologic disorders experience no unusual creative powers. They face a degenerative clinical course and early death. But the spark of genius, even when ignited by illness, may shed light on unexplored areas of the mind, although how the brain supports the creative process remains as much a mystery as π.

Mathematicians and artists alike have turned to repetition and exquisite detail in their search for perfection. And so have public health researchers. Exhaustive reporting and integration of surveillance data can identify specimens for genetic analysis and clarify variants associated with susceptibility to central nervous system disease.

Bibliography

Bovers M, Hagen F, Kuramae EE, et al. AIDS patient death caused by novel *Cryptococcus neoformans* × *C. gattii* hybrid. *Emerg Infect Dis.* 2008;14:1105–1108.

Ceyhan M, Yildirim I, Balmer P, et al. A prospective study of etiology of childhood acute bacterial meningitis, Turkey. *Emerg Infect Dis.* 2008;14:1089–1096.

Crawford DC, Zimmer SM, Morin CA, et al. Integrating host genomics with surveillance for invasive bacterial diseases. *Emerg Infect Dis.* 2008;14:1138–1140.

Jourdan-Morhange H. *Ravel et nous*. Geneva, Switzerland: Ed. du Milieu du Monde; 1945.

Kavanaugh P. *Music of the Great Composers*. Grand Rapids, MI: Zondervan; 1996.

Orenstein A. *The Ballets of Maurice Ravel: Creation and Interpretation*. Burlington, VT: Ashgate; 1991.

Pérez-Osorio CE, Zavala-Velázquez JE, León JJA, et al. *Rickettsia felis* as emergent global threat for humans. *Emerg Infect Dis.* 2008;14:1019–1023.

Seeley WW, Matthews BR, Crawford RK, et al. Unravelling Boléro: progressive aphasia, transmodal creativity and the right posterior neocortex. *Brain.* 2008;131:39–49.

EMERGING

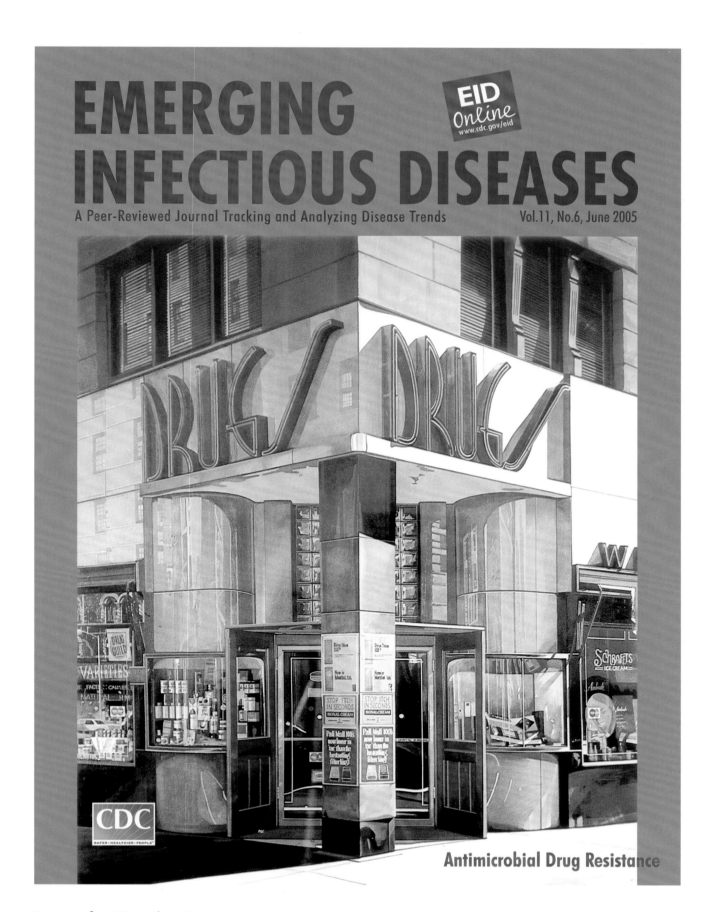

EID Online
www.cdc.gov/eid

INFECTIOUS DISEASES

A Peer-Reviewed Journal Tracking and Analyzing Disease Trends

Vol.11, No.6, June 2005

Antimicrobial Drug Resistance

DRUGS, MICROBES, AND ANTIMICROBIAL RESISTANCE

"If America is to produce great painters," wrote great American painter Thomas Eakins (1844–1916), young artists should "remain in America to peer deeper into the heart of American life." Eakins traveled abroad, where he became familiar with the work of 19th-century greats Gustave Courbet, Édouard Manet, and Edgar Degas, but returned home to become a master of realism whose exactness and precision influenced many 20th-century American painters, one of them Richard Estes.

Estes, a native of Kewanee, Illinois, grew up in Chicago and attended the city's famed Art Institute. Upon graduation in 1956, he moved to New York to pursue a career in graphic design as freelance illustrator for magazines and advertising agencies. In the next 10 years, he crossed over to fine art and had his first exhibit around 1968.

An admirer of Eakins, Estes peered deeply into the American cityscape for a new style of art, true not only to his native culture but also to his times. This style evoked the traditions of *trompe l'oeil* (fooling the eye through photographic illusion) and of 17th-century Dutch painting to create a contemporary version of reality. "When you look at a scene or an object you tend to scan it. Your eye travels around and over things. As your eye moves the vanishing point moves," Estes said in an interview. "To have one vanishing point or perfect camera perspective is not realistic."

Drawing from his surroundings rather than the imagination, Estes used photography to collect images or frozen moments of light on surfaces to complement his own recollection of places and objects. He did not reproduce photographic scenes. From multiple images, he selected certain elements, abstracting and arranging them to best advantage, exaggerating angles and omitting extraneous detail. This innovative perception and composition of visual reality came to be called superrealism or photorealism, a new art movement co-founded by Estes in the late 1960s.

Photorealists, many of them influenced by Estes, painted varied images, portraits as well as landscapes, in exquisite detail. Their subjects were diners and storefronts, gumball machines, neon lights, pickup trucks, and other trappings of 1970s American life. Estes was captivated by the contemporary urban landscape, particularly of New York, where he has lived much of his life, although he has also worked in Chicago, Venice, and Paris. One in a long line of artists to know and paint New York, he has worked in terms that seem architectural in their emphasis on structure and design and created of this landscape a veritable visual spectacle for posterity. Buildings, bridges, traffic patterns, city curbs were manipulated and transformed from commonplace scenes into grand theater, much more intense and "real" on canvas than ever in their own existence.

Yet, even as he has created an archivist's treasure of Downtown Manhattan and Manhattan's Upper West Side, Estes is not interested in nostalgia or future archaeologic records. And as much as he has been compared with 18th-century Italian artists (e.g., Canaletto), who painted palaces, piazzas, and canals, he is not interested in urban scenery for its beauty or underlying social commentary. He paints for the sake of painting, usually with acrylic color overlaid with oils, lovingly reinventing the scenes he explores.

"Daily life has a reputation for being banal, uninteresting, boring somehow. It strikes me that daily life is baffling, mysterious, and unfathomable." These are the words of George Segal, Estes's contemporary and colleague, who saw magic in the mundane. Estes walks around the streets of New York until something catches his eye. He returns to the scene on weekends or evenings when the streets are deserted to take photos. Later in his studio, he reconstructs what he saw and collected, in a scene become more fiction than reality. Unlike Segal's work, which witnesses a moment of human existence, Estes's witnesses the moment itself and celebrates its visual presence with clarity and exactness.

In his meticulous reconstructions, Estes eliminates clutter, shadows, people—as if by scrubbing the scene, he can extract its essence and verify its existence. Singling out the structural, he elaborates on it from multiple angles, under a uniformly glaring light, and produces a sharp image much more compelling and deliberate than any captured by the naked eye. In the process, a perfectly dull building, an anonymous row of telephone booths, a street corner become arresting and memorable.

In *DRUGS*, Estes's penetrating eye examines an icon of contemporary city life, the corner drugstore. Expertly cropped, central, and direct, the structure invites inspection on several levels: storefront and curb, window displays, and nearby buildings mirrored on shiny surfaces. A prominent column, neatly plastered with ads, blocks visual access to the interior, even with the entrance doors propped wide open against the sidewalk. The windows upstairs are shut. Elaborate glass facets and distortions of light restrict the viewer to the exterior.

Intentionally or not, Estes's drugstore, with its pristine appearance, reflects more than the block across the street. A cornerstone in the life of the city and the development of modern medicine, the institution it represents has held tricks of the medical trade, from camphor to penicillin to telithromycin. This shining apothecary symbolizes human efforts to improve health and control disease, efforts often stymied by the complexity of the task.

Not unlike artists, scientists in disease control seek order in a complicated universe. With their powerful microscopes, they too focus on the details as they construct clear, artificially uncluttered versions of a crowded microbial world. Singling out microbes that cause disease, scientists scrutinize, isolate them, and neutralize their effects on human health through powerful drugs. For their part, the microbes expel, modify, or exclude the drugs, prompting a new cycle of drug development, also destined for obsolescence. Antimicrobial drug resistance, begun with the first antimicrobial drug, threatens the single-microbe approach to disease control and the venerable institution Estes immortalized in *DRUGS*.

Bibliography

Arthur J. *Richard Estes: The Urban Landscape*. Boston, MA: Museum of Fine Arts and New York Graphic Society; 1978.

Bonito VA. Richard Estes and the contemporary American realists; http://www.artregister.com/; accessed March 2, 2005.

Cohen D, ed. A dialogue between Gregory J. Peterson and Richard Estes; http://www.artcritical.com; accessed March 2, 2005.

Kimball R. Master craftsman. Available at: http://www.artchive.com/artchive/E/eakins.html; accessed April 25, 2013.

Meisel LK. *Photorealism*. New York, NY: Harry N. Abrams; 1980.

Segal G. American still life; http://www.pbs.org/georgesegal/index; accessed March 1, 2005.

The story of modern art: Richard Estes. http://hirshhorn.si.edu/; accessed March 2, 2005.

Weber JT, Courvalin P. An emptying quiver: antimicrobial drugs and resistance. *Emerg Infect Dis.* 2005;11:791–793.

Climate, Weather, Ecosystems

*H*unters in the Snow was created during a frigid period known as the Little Ice Age, the second part of the 16th century. Glaciers were advancing rapidly in Greenland, Iceland, Scandinavia, and the Alps; the arctic pack ice extended so far south that Eskimos were reported landing their kayaks in Scotland; and large tracts of land at higher altitudes were abandoned. With this famed snowscape, Flemish artist Pieter Bruegel the Elder (1525–1569) started a new genre by painting as many as seven winter landscapes in 2 years, immortalizing the gloom and desolation in expansive olive gray scenes of thick snow. His hunters in the snow, crouched figures moving with difficulty against the wind, appeared very small and unimportant in the winter vista. Other villagers who came out to play in what seems an ice-skating opportunity, a frozen lake in the background, seemed speckles of no consequence. Nature was clearly in control.

Nature is still in control when it comes to climate and weather. Arctic communities are again facing health and economic challenges because of melting permafrost, flooding, and storm surges, which are progressively destroying village sanitation and drinking water infrastructures and are paving the way for outbreaks of food- and water-borne diseases and respiratory infections. Fred Machetanz's *Quest for Avuk* explores the plight of Arctic populations in the United States and Canada, whose lives have changed because of warmer weather. No longer isolated by thick ice and still unaccustomed to thawing conditions, they have become vulnerable to emerging infections. A *Festival Banner, Nepal, 17th century*, confirms this connection. When the glaciers began to melt, removing barriers between Nepal and the outside world, travel reached the remotest peaks and with it sex trafficking, which has been linked with the spread of HIV across South Asia. Sex-trafficked women and girls from Nepal who are infected with HIV are more likely than those not infected to also have syphilis and hepatitis B.

Climate fluctuations influence the replication and movement of pathogens and their carriers, as well as the ecology and human behavior. Infections caused by mosquito-borne viruses are strongly influenced by weather conditions or display a seasonality that indicates such influence. A warming trend may expand or shift areas favorable to mosquito breeding. Changes in levels of precipitation and humidity affect the range and survivability of both carriers and pathogens. The incidence of West Nile virus disease is seasonal in the temperate zones of North America, Europe, and the Mediterranean Basin, with peak activity from July through October. In the United States, the transmission season has lengthened as the virus has moved south; in 2003, onset of human illness began as late as December, and in 2004, as early as April.

West Nile virus was first detected in the Western Hemisphere in 1999 during an outbreak of encephalitis in New York City. Over the next 5 years, the virus spread across the continental United States, north into Canada, and south into the Caribbean Islands and Latin America, primarily by the bite of mosquitoes, which get it by feeding on infected birds. Intensity of transmission to humans depends on the abundance and feeding patterns of infected mosquitoes. Local ecology and behavior contribute too as they influence human exposure to these pests. On one of the covers in this chapter, Emily Carr's emblematic *Big Raven*, a large crow reminiscent of totem symbolizes passed plagues in the community of its artistic origins. It also stands for birds of the crow family, whose deaths usually precede West Nile virus infections in humans in North America and elsewhere. The predicament of these birds, prophetic as it is of human deaths, informs the ecology and dispersal of disease.

Interaction between disease vectors, animal reservoirs, microbes, and humans allows environmental changes to influence transmission dynamics. Many of the factors that affect the abundance, survival, activity, or feeding behavior of vectors also affect the reproduction, survival, and abundance of animal reservoirs. Elevated rainfall creates new breeding habitats for mosquitoes and increases mosquito population density. The same factors can affect human behavior or exposure to infection by influencing outdoor activities, housing, the quality and quantity of food, and agricultural or other uses of the environment. Paul Gauguin's *I Raro te Oviri* (*Under the Pandanus*), set in the tropical paradise that inspired his best art, invites inspection of arthropod-borne infections rampant in the hot and humid environment.

In the landmark outbreak of hantavirus pulmonary syndrome in the southwestern United States in 1993, the causative hantavirus may have been present in mouse populations in the region for a long time, but an unusually mild and wet winter and spring led to increases in rodent populations in the spring and summer and thus to greater opportunities for people to come in contact with infected rodents and with the virus. This weather anomaly may have been part of a broader pattern responsible for outbreaks of similar disease in Europe at approximately the same time. In South America, several outbreaks of hantavirus infections have been linked to forest clearance and growth of rodent populations in new grasslands.

Other weather anomalies, such as extraordinary storms or other disasters that result in breakdown of public health measures, are behind the reemergence of infections that might have otherwise been under control or entirely eliminated. Katsushika Hokusai's *The Great Wave off Kanagawa* offers a glimpse of weather-related catastrophe of the kind tossed on coastal populations. When the waters are stirred, communities crumble. In the aftermath comes infectious disease, originating in the disruption and lingering for lack of hygienic conditions and adequate medical care.

To be transported over relatively long distances from one host to another, many microbes must by borne passively through moving air or water. Some pathogenic microbes, such as those causing coccidioidomycosis, are picked up from the soil and carried by dry, dusty winds. Others, like those causing cryptosporidiosis, may be washed by heavy rains into reservoirs of drinking water. Community water resources are frequently associated with disease emergence. Breakdowns in water treatment have resulted in large waterborne disease outbreaks. Water that is inadequately treated can transmit infectious bacteria, viruses, and parasites. Inadequate filtration caused the 1993 outbreak of cryptosporidiosis, a parasitic disease, in Milwaukee, Wisconsin, where more than 400,000 residents became ill. Frank Day's *Konkow Maidu (The Water Test)* amplifies the microbial population to warn of the threat lurking in the water.

The cover images in this chapter allude to the impact of climate change on host–parasite interactions, animal population dynamics, and human health. Alexis Rockman's *Manifesting Ecologic and Microbial Connections* offers the panoramic view of a landscape gone wrong under extreme climate and ecosystem stresses. This extraordinary artistic vision stresses the symbiotic nature of emergence and warns against complacency.

Bibliography

Kemp M. Looking at the face of the Earth. *Nature* 2008;456(18):876.

Williams WC. The hunter in the snow. Available at: http://english.emory.edu/classes/paintings&poems/hunters.html. Accessed June 4, 2013.

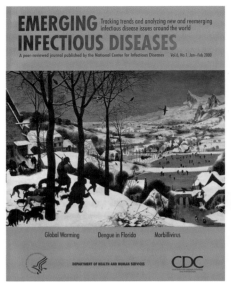

Global Warming; http://dx.doi.org/10.3201/eid0601.AC0601

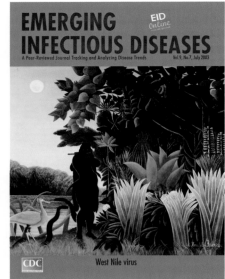

West Nile Virus; http://dx.doi.org/10.3201/eid0907.AC0907

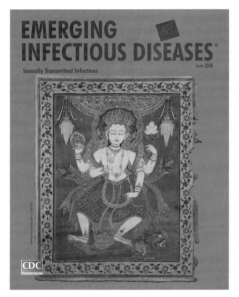

Sexually Transmitted Infections; http://dx.doi.org/10.3201/eid1406.AC1406

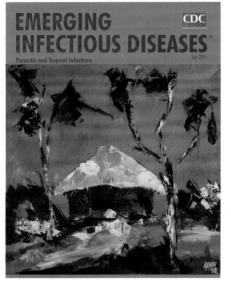

Parasitic and Tropical Infections; http://dx.doi.org/10.3201/eid1707.AC1707

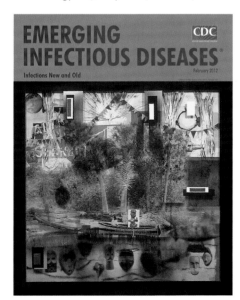

Infections New and Old; http://dx.doi.org/10.3201/eid1802.AC1802

EMERGING
INFECTIOUS DISEASES®

EID Online
www.cdc.gov/eid

January 2008

International Polar Year

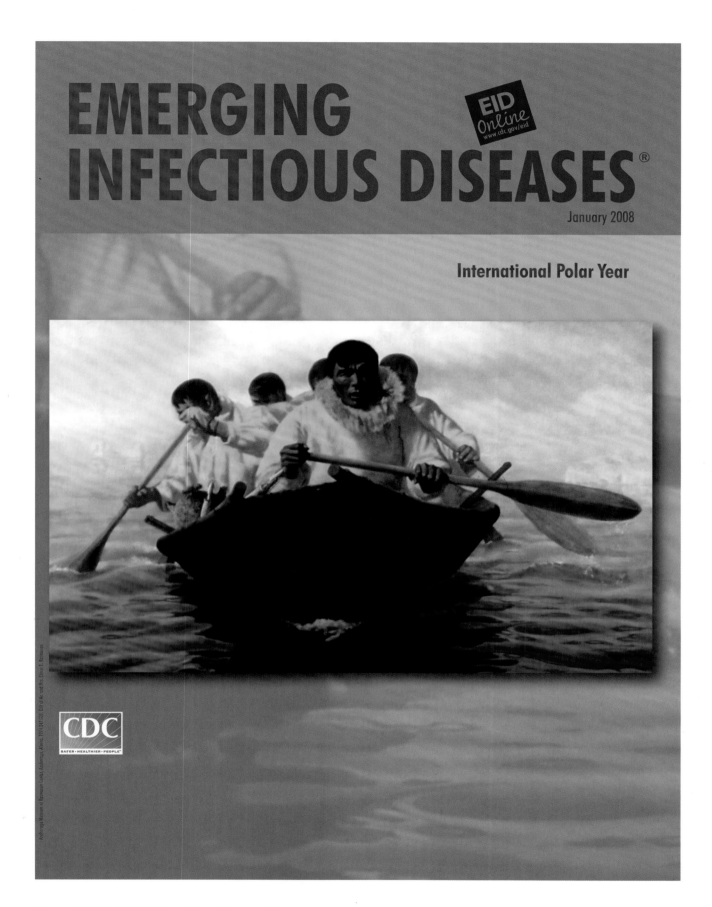

CDC
SAFER·HEALTHIER·PEOPLE™

I AM BUT MAD NORTH-NORTHWEST: WHEN THE WIND IS SOUTHERLY I KNOW A HAWK FROM A HANDSAW[1]

"The true north strong and choked with ice," wrote Canadian poet Al Purdy, about the Arctic. "The sea . . . was like the concentrated essence of all the blue that ever was; I could feel that blue seep into me and all my innards change colour. And the icebergs! They were shimmery lace and white brocade, and they became my standard for the word beauty." Purdy's thrill at drifting with "the tides on Cumberland Sound and its blue fiord, [where] bergs and growlers are always in sight, even at the height of summer" echoes the experience of many who visit the North; among them, Fred Machetanz, painter of iconic Alaska.

A native of Kenton, Ohio, educated at Ohio State University, the American Academy of Art in Chicago, and the Arts Students League in New York, Fred Machetanz ventured to Unalakleet, a tiny fishing village on the Bering Sea, in 1935 to visit his uncle. Captivated by the landscape, he moved there to celebrate it in his work for years to come. "I was just nuts about Alaska."

Artists have long traveled to the icy North. During the 18th and 19th centuries, as part of explorations, they documented discoveries and sought adventure and new cultures. John Webber, official painter for Captain James Cook's voyage (1776–1780), produced countless expertly painted records. By the end of European exploration and after the purchase of Alaska in 1867 from the Russians, travel increased. Naturalists and conservationists, John Burroughs, John Muir, and others, reported on their visits to the glaciers. North American artists, among them Eustace Ziegler, Ted Lambert, Sidney Laurence, and Jules Dahlager, migrated to paint their romantic vision of "the last frontier" with its pristine wilderness and sparse inhabitants close to the land. Some of these visitors became the best landscape painters of the day. The art of Alaska's own populations, a long and rich tradition, was influenced by the onslaught of imported forms.

Much history of the Eskimo culture of North America in early 20th century comes to us from the work of Danish anthropologist Knud Rasmussen, whose expedition crossed North America from east of Baffin Land to Alaska and across the Bering Straight to Siberia. He lived to report conditions more inclement and dangerous for humans than nearly anywhere else in the world. "Cold and mosquitoes, / these two pests / come never together," goes the Iglulik song, "I lay me down on the ice, / Lay me down on the snow and the ice, / Till my teeth fall chattering."

The relationship between humans and the physical world is widely explored in Inuit poetry. "We fear the weather spirit of earth, which we must fight against to wrest our food from land and sea. We fear Sila [the weather]." Locals and sourdoughs of a bygone era under these extreme conditions, their rules for life and survival from snowstorm to snowstorm, the majestic surroundings and wildlife became Machetanz's work—during the early years, in books, photographs, movies, and lectures; then exclusively in paintings. He set up his easel opposite

---

1 William Shakespeare, *Hamlet* (2.2.276–277).

the windows of his tiny cabin near Palmer and started to re-create the surroundings. Over seven decades, he exhibited widely, built a reputation, and became one of Alaska's most beloved artists. "If anyone viewing my work has felt the beauty, the thrills and the fascination I have known in Alaska, then I have succeeded in what I set out to do."

Though close to the artists of Alaska's romantic era, Machetanz lived the life he painted. He embraced the wilderness, "Why that land that they want back there ain't fit for nobody but goats, writers and artists" was the official opinion on the space staked out for his cabin. He joined a whaling crew, paddled his own umiak, drove dog sleds. If he painted an Athabascan woman with a birch bark baby carrier, he commissioned a carrier. "That's why we have these beautiful artifacts we've collected, which are made to scale, and made by experts, the natives who know them." He could "take a model and rotate it in the sunlight and get the light and shade on it."

The art editor of Scribner's once joked about a Machetanz painting, "You've put a cherry colored head on that Eskimo." The painter corrected him, "If you see an Eskimo under a golden pink sun, you're going to see a red exactly like that. . . . People don't realize the colors that we get here. And then we have a longer chance to look at those colors" because of the long hours of daylight in the summer and late spring.

As a young man, Machetanz visited Maxfield Parrish, then probably the most famous American artist; "hardly a home in America existed that didn't have a Maxfield Parrish print." He drove to Cornish, New Hampshire, to meet him, and they became friends for life. "I have always admired the art of Maxfield Parrish and a lot of the early painters of the Renaissance . . . Vermeer and Titian and those. They used a technique . . . where they first, on the canvas or board . . . painted the entire painting in one color—white . . . then . . . layers of transparent color, which you could look through and eventually get the final result. It's like putting a blue glass and a red glass over a white surface, and you could look through the blue and the red and you could see a purple, but it would be a transparent purple and quite different from an opaque purple of pigment." This laborious technique is credited for the chill northern intensity of Machetanz's paintings: "each layer has to be dry before I put on another layer, and my paintings contain six to eight layers of paint and varnish, and the only way I could dry them was by the sun or the stove."

Quest for Avuk captures a theme of everyday life. Eskimo men paddle an umiak, a lightweight skin boat of the Arctic, searching for Avuk, likely a walrus (*ayvuq* [Central Siberian Yupik], *aiviq* [Inupiaq]). The men in camouflage kuspuks of cotton canvas over their parkas wear a look of intense concentration. A rifle, a toggling harpoon, and a sealskin float are visible from the side. The lithe vessel gliding noiselessly on the frigid waters allows immediate access to the hunt beneath the surface: seals, walruses, whales; in back, ice always in the invisible horizon.

"When I get home / With a catch that does not suffice, / I usually say / It was the fish / That failed—/ Up the stream." A hard stormy winter, when the caribou left and the seals were hard to find, could spell starvation for Machetanz's subjects, early Eskimo communities, isolated, completely dependent on traditional sources of sustenance, lashed by weather. "Life is so with us that we are never surprised . . . that someone has starved to death. We are so used to it . . . They cannot help it, it is not their fault, it is either sila [the weather] or persaq [blizzard] or to'nraq [evil spirit, i.e., sickness]."

"I have only my song, / Though it too is slipping from me." Arctic populations in the United States and Canada now live largely in settled communities no longer completely dependent on walrus and fish. Long adapted to isolation and affected by infections linked to climate and culture, they are now also vulnerable to emerging plagues. Back in the 1980s, in his "Trees at the Arctic Circle," Al Purdy contemplated the strength of these trees: "And you know it occurs to me / about 2 feet under / those roots must touch permafrost / ice that remains ice forever / and they use it for their nourishment / use death to remain alive." Now permafrost is melting. Heavily geared for ice, Arctic populations are facing yet another bout of rough weather, a warming trend. And unlike Shakespeare's hero, they have no need to feign madness.

Bibliography

Oral history with Fred Machetanz. 1988. Located at: UAA/APU Archives and Special Collections Department, Anchorage, AK.

Parkinson AJ. The international polar year 2007–2008, an opportunity to focus on infectious diseases in Arctic regions. *Emerg Infect Dis.* 2008;14:1–3.

Purdy A. *Starting from Ameliasburgh: The Collected Prose of Al Purdy.* Solecki S, ed. Madeira Park, Canada: Harbour; 1995.

Purdy A. To see the shore: a preface. In: *The Collected Poems of Al Purdy* by Purdy ed. Russell Brown. Toronto, Canada: McClelland and Stewart; 1986.

Rasmussen K. *Intellectual Culture of the Iglulik Eskimos.* Copenhagen, Denmark: Thule Report; 1929.

Woodward KE. *Painting Alaska.* Anchorage, AK: Alaska Geographic Society; 2000.

Woodward KE. *A Northern Adventure: The Art of Fred Machetanz.* Augusta, GA: Morris Communications; 2004.

EMERGING
INFECTIOUS DISEASES®

February 2011

Influenza

Hamburger Kunsthalle, Hamburg, Germany/The Bridgeman Art Library

THE ICY REALM OF THE RIME

The "taciturn man from the North" is how his contemporaries described Caspar David Friedrich, referring to his melancholy, or in his own words, his "dreadful weariness," especially in later years. Loneliness pervaded his work as well as his life, which was marred by early deaths in the family—of his mother when he was 7 and several siblings, among them, a young brother, who drowned in a frozen lake, according to some, trying to rescue him.

Friedrich was born in Greifswald, then Swedish Pomerania, on the Baltic coast of Germany, the son of a candle maker and soap boiler in a family of 10 children. As a youth he studied with architect and painter Johann Gottfried Quistorp but later moved to Copenhagen to attend the Academy, one of the leading centers of art in Europe, and eventually settled in Dresden. His training in the neoclassical tradition relied on extensive preliminary studies, drawings, and sketches to depict the physical world and is reflected in the disciplined quality of all his works. But while his landscapes were always actual studies of nature, they were more than a representation of nature.

This man, who according to his contemporaries discovered "the tragedy of landscape" and gained by it fame in his own time, soon embraced an untested individual approach to painting, despite a lingering attachment to the systematic techniques of his training. "The artist should paint not only what he sees before him, but also what he sees within him," he wrote. This belief was rooted in his view of nature as a subject itself worthy of study, imbued with spiritual qualities and portrayed entirely without human presence, not as backdrop but as protagonist. His interest was not in the beauty of nature alone but in what the romantics called the sublime—powerful natural phenomena: snowstorms, impenetrable fog, impassable mountains—generating conflicted feelings of wonder and helplessness, which he could sense and capture with symbols and allegorical elements.

Viewing and presenting the landscape in an entirely new way was Friedrich's main innovation. He turned the mountains, forests, and vistas of northern German countryside in the times of Beethoven, Schubert, and Goethe into romantic icons, painting them at all times of night and day, around Dresden and the River Elbe, especially in the moonlight and sunlight or covered with mist. "Close your bodily eye so that you may see your picture first with the spiritual eye. Then bring to the light of day that which you have seen in the darkness so that it may react upon others from the outside inwards," he wrote in his notes on aesthetics in 1830. Therefore, his winter landscapes were not about life in the winter but about winter itself, stark, still, desolate, where "no man has yet set his foot."

Despite early fame and a prolific career, Friedrich lost ground in his mature years and fell into poverty, becoming the "most solitary of the solitary." Bare trees and stumps populated with ravens and owls near graveyards and ruins filled his works, expressing the passage of time and his own state of mind. But these late paintings also explored a mystical approach, one abandoning the self to reach an intuitive understanding of physical phenomena. This period's frisson of the sublime was later adopted by Hollywood directors to show horror, trepidation, and other emotions caused by human inadequacy against the overpowering forces of nature.

The Polar Sea expresses Friedrich's mature vision, which, far ahead of his times, was not well received. The painting was inspired by William Parry's arctic expedition of 1819–20, a venture filled with opportunities for symbolic interpretation. The artist seized these to build a monument to nature's triumph over human efforts to conquer it. The tiny image of the ship, inscribed HMS Griber, against a mount of ice, signals the insignificance of human enterprise. Frightful shards jut into the steel gray sky atop solid slabs of ice that form a frigid grave over what human presence might have existed before the wreck and builds a wall between the viewer and the ship.

Another leading romantic, Samuel Taylor Coleridge wrote prolifically about imagery deep with symbolism. In "The Rime of the Ancient Mariner," he offered his version of beautiful and ominous nature, set in a metaphysical world. Among the many influences on this poem were vivid accounts by arctic explorers. Like Friedrich, Coleridge was fascinated by their travails, which he immortalized. Here is the Mariner's ship in the grip of polar ice: "And now there came both mist and snow, / And it grew wondrous cold: / The ice, mast high, came floating by / As green as emerald. . . . / The ice, was here, the ice was there, / the ice was all around: / It cracked and growled, and roared and howled, / Like noises in a swound!/"

The "rime" in the world of both Friedrich and Coleridge is symbolic of the sublime world of nature. At once fascinating and terrifying, it changes forms: water, ice, mist—taxing visual awareness, toying with the artist, challenging the scientist, tempting the poet. When European mariners were searching for the Northwest Passage, formidable polar ice lay between them and navigation. The routing was lined with myth and uncertainty, hunger, and scurvy. How times have changed! Now instead of the powerful solidity of ice, we fear instead its fragility as the polar ice cap threatens to melt into the sea, exposing among other puzzles the dynamic evolutionary interface between human viruses and the ice that can preserve and protect them for thousands of years. What remains constant is nature's upper hand.

In 1918, as explorers were plowing their way into the Arctic, other events were also making history. World War I was coming to a close, yet weary humanity already had a new serious concern, one that was to cause more deaths around the globe than this and future wars combined. The public health emergency spread widely in the fall of the year. Only 3 days after taking sail, the Forsete arrived at Longyearbyen, a tiny village in Spitsbergen Island, Svalbard, Norway, north of the Arctic Circle. An outbreak of flu had broken out on the ship caused as it turned out by an extraordinarily potent strain that would become known as Spanish Flu. Many passengers, young miners, were hospitalized and over the next few weeks, seven of them died. Their bodies, containing the deadliest flu virus the world has ever known, were buried in the local cemetery, 800 miles from the North Pole.

Almost eight decades later, a similar grave in Alaska permafrost held valuable clues about the Spanish Flu pandemic. Unlike the one concocted in Friedrich's imagination, this grave was not a monument to human failure. Its contents enabled RNA sequencing of much of the 1918 virus. As the ice melts, more secrets of the great pandemic may see the light of day, guiding present flu prevention activities. Moreover, other illnesses become endemic in new areas as a result of changes in climate. Tick-borne encephalitis seems to be moving northward in Europe and shifting upward on 84 mountains apparently influenced by such changes. Frozen solid or melting fast, sublime nature rules.

Bibliography

Altmann M, Fiebig L, Soyka J, et al. Severe cases of pandemic (H1N1) 2009 in children, Germany. *Emerg Infect Dis.* 2011;17:184–190.

Duncan K. *Hunting the 1918 Flu: One Scientist's Search for a Killer Virus.* Toronto, Canada: University of Toronto Press; 2003.

Hofmann W. *Caspar David Friedrich.* London, England: Thames and Hudson; 2001.

Jääskeläinen AE, Tonteri E, Sironen T, et al. Tick-borne encephalitis virus, Finnish Lapland. *Emerg Infect Dis.* 2011;17:323–324.

Schrauwen EJ, Herfst S, Chutinimitkul S, et al. Possible increased pathogenicity of pandemic (H1N1) 2009 influenza virus upon reassortment. *Emerg Infect Dis.* 2011;17:198–206.

Siegel L. *Caspar David Friedrich and the Age of German Romanticism.* Boston, MA: Branden Books; 1978.

Taubenberger JK, Reid AH, Lourens RM, et al. Characterization of the 1918 influenza polymerase gene. *Nature.* 2005;437:889–893.

Vaughan W. *Friedrich.* London, England: Phaidon Press; 2004.

EMERGING

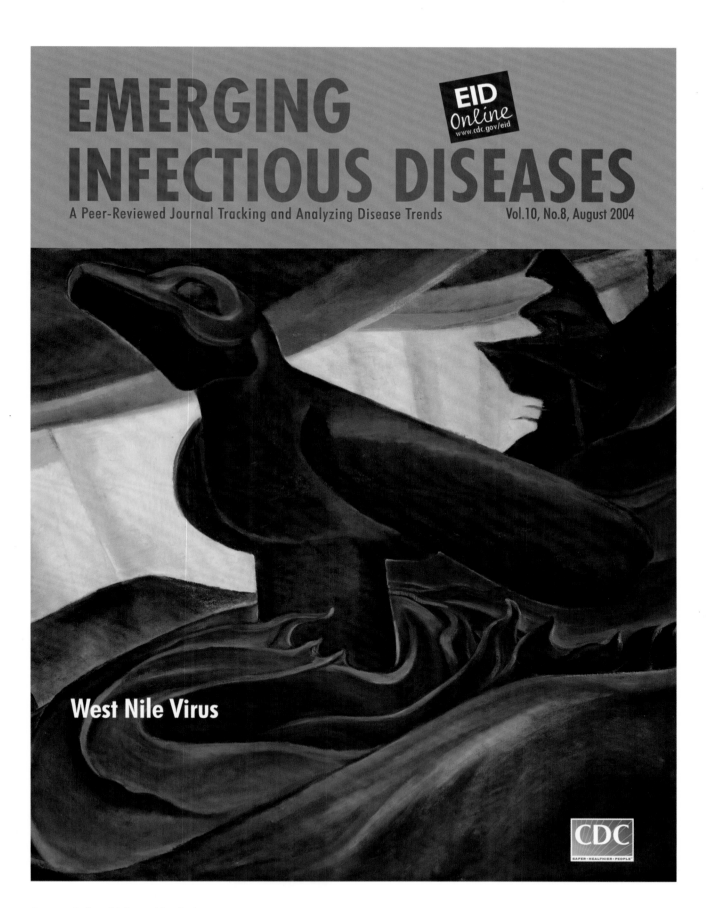

EID
Online
www.cdc.gov/eid

INFECTIOUS DISEASES

A Peer-Reviewed Journal Tracking and Analyzing Disease Trends

Vol.10, No.8, August 2004

West Nile Virus

CDC
SAFER·HEALTHIER·PEOPLE™

"Prophet!" said I, "thing of evil!—prophet still, if bird or devil!
Whether tempter sent, or whether tempest tossed thee here ashore,
Desolate, yet all undaunted, on this desert land enchanted—
On this home by horror haunted—tell me—tell me I implore!"
Is there—is there balm in Gilead?—tell me—tell me I implore!"[2]

"Not far from the house sat a great wooden raven mounted on a rather low pole; his wings were flattened to his sides. . . . His mate . . . had rotted away long ago, leaving him moss-grown, dilapidated and alone . . . these two great birds had been set, one on either side of the doorway of a big house that had been full of dead Indians who had died during a smallpox epidemic. Bursting growth . . . grew up round the . . . raven, sheltering him from the tearing winds now that he was old and rotting." wrote Emily Carr in *Klee Wyck*, the best-selling book of short stories about her many visits to Native villages near Victoria, Canada, where she was born.

Artist, author, and passionate advocate of trees and birds, Carr drew inspiration and focus from decaying aboriginal artifacts that littered the wilderness of her beloved British Columbia. Many of her works seem haunted by these artifacts' legacy of epidemics and death. With a "smothering darkness," descended perhaps from her own Anglo-Victorian culture's fear of the primeval forest, she conveyed the frailty of human efforts against the power of the woods and the spirits in them.

Carr pursued an artistic career from age 16 and attended the California School of Design in San Francisco. She taught art; traveled to England, France, and the wilds of Canada's Pacific Coast in search of personal style; and exhibited widely, in spite of financial constraints and ill health from heart disease and frequent bouts of depression. Her dedication to the natural world and her belief in the mystical and spiritual connection between all things culminated during the latter part of her life (1933–1936) in landscapes of "exceptional spontaneity and expressiveness."

The late 19th century witnessed sweeping cultural changes. Existing values were questioned in science, philosophy, and the arts, at the individual and social levels. This was the era of, among countless greats, Robert Koch, Louis Pasteur, Charles Darwin, Marie Curie, Albert Einstein, Fredrich Nietzsche, Sigmund Freud, George Eliot, Walt Whitman, and Mary Cassatt. Artists were moving away from descriptive likeness toward visual impression of objects. During her travels to Europe, Carr explored modernism and pondered its "big ideas" in the context of the "big land" of her childhood, adopting new styles, transcending her own experience, creating potent landscapes for the world.

Like fellow North American artists Georgia O'Keeffe and Frida Kahlo, Carr turned for authenticity to nature and to her own and Native cultures. The wilderness of British Columbia and southern Alaska and the work of Pacific Coast communities roused her artistic imagination. She came to view nature as anthropomorphic and

---

2 Edgar Allan Poe, "The Raven."

trees, stars, rocks, and all natural forms as symbolic reality with which she could identify—once, in a rare self-portrait, she painted herself in the form of a tree.

Carr continued to paint decaying tribal artifacts as she experimented with modern techniques. And by adapting the structuring influence of cubism to paintings of Pacific Coast tribal art, she did more than preserve this art from extinction. She brought history full circle by reviving and reformulating artifacts whose kin, the tribal art of Africa and South Pacific, had greatly influenced the development of cubism in France.

Big Raven evolved from the watercolor image of a Haida totem pole Carr had painted at Cumshewa, Queen Charlotte Islands, almost 20 years earlier. "I want to bring a great loneliness to this canvas and a haunting broodiness, quiet and powerful," the artist wrote in her journal. Broodiness notwithstanding, *Big Raven* is full of energy and movement. The sky and landscape are sculptured, as solid and heavy as the raven itself, yet their interlocking elements are spirited. They heave and swell, their scalloped edges undulating in a powerful swirl around the massive bird.

This remnant of a vibrant household struck down by the plague of its time stands a lonely symbol of passing plagues in Carr's green sea of anthropomorphic nature. Perched low, impassive, silent, and seemingly unmoved, it feigns obscurity and anonymity, but the upward avian thrust, grave countenance, and ghastly glare label it prophet of doom.

A single bird like Carr's lonely oracle sends proper warning. A population of birds in distress or dying is a far more useful sentinel; watchful tracking of their predicament informs the ecology and dispersal of disease. Animals turn sentinels as their deaths presage human illness on the epidemic curve. Dying prairie dogs signal human plague in the American Southwest. Horses dying of eastern equine encephalomyelitis point to increased spread of virus in a community. When an "Old World epizootic strain," West Nile virus, made its way across North America, from the Atlantic to the Pacific Coasts, from Canada into tropical regions and the Caribbean, unexplained avian deaths sometimes occurred weeks before human West Nile virus encephalitis cases. And dying birds of the crow family, including ravens, foretold human infection in the New World as they likely did in ancient Babylon.

Bibliography

Beloved land, the world of Emily Carr (Introduction by Robin Lawrence). Vancouver/Toronto, Canada: Douglas & McIntyre; 1996.

Carr E. *Klee Wyck*. Vancouver, Canada: Douglas & McIntyre; 2003.

Centers for Disease Control and Prevention. Plague prevention. Available at: http://www.cdc.gov/plague/.

County of Los Angeles, Public Health. Field manual of wildlife diseases. Available at: http://www.lapublichealth.org/vet/guides/vetzooman.htm; accessed April 25, 2013.

Emily Carr biography; http://collections.ic.gc.ca; accessed May 13, 2004.

Marr JS, Calisher CH. Alexander the Great and West Nile virus encephalitis. *Emerg Infect Dis.* 2003;9:1599–1603.

National Museum of Women in the Arts; http://www.nmwa.org/pubs; accessed May 13, 2004.

Reisen W, Lothrop H, Chiles R, et al. West Nile virus in California. *Emerg Infect Dis.* 2004;10:1369–1378.

Vol 10, No 4, April 2004

DEPARTMENT OF
HEALTH & HUMAN SERVICES
Public Health Service
Centers for Disease Control and Prevention (CDC)
Atlanta, GA 30333

Official Business
Penalty for Private Use $300

Return Service Requested

EMERGING INFECTIOUS DISEASES

A Peer-Reviewed Journal Tracking and Analyzing Disease Trends

Vol.10, No.4, April 2004

EID
Online
www.cdc.gov/eid

EMERGING INFECTIOUS DISEASES

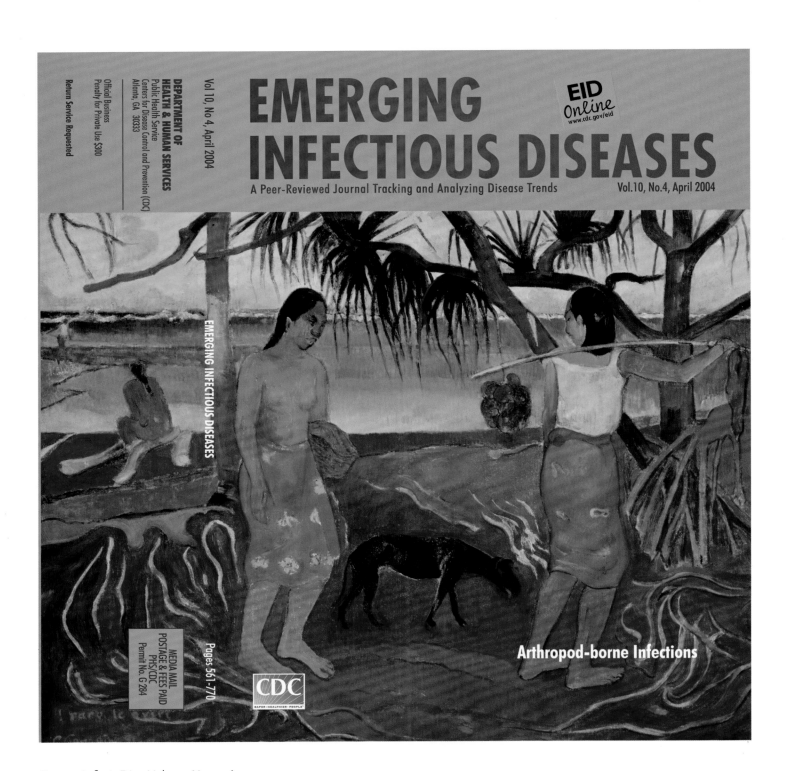

Arthropod-borne Infections

MEDIA MAIL
POSTAGE & FEES PAID
PHS/CDC
Permit No. G 284

Pages 561-770

CDC

TROUBLE IN PARADISE

"Between me and the sky there was nothing except the high frail roof of the pandanus leaves, where the lizards have their nests," wrote Paul Gauguin in the autobiographical account of his first visit to Tahiti. *Under the Pandanus* was painted shortly after Gauguin arrived on the islands in search of his famed reprieve from Western civilization.

Like many of his contemporaries, Gauguin became disillusioned with industrialized society whose intense focus on material gain seemed to strip life of its spiritual essence. Crushed under the yoke of familial responsibility, bewildered by the prosaic rules of art dealing, and stifled by societal constraints, Gauguin imagined a life uncluttered by the tedium of survival. He longed for a different world, one with just enough depth to sustain his most basic needs. Flat and two dimensional, this world would be filled with vibrant color and would celebrate the human spirit long lost under oppressive layers of cultural complexity and control.

While many rebel against civilization and espouse notions of an unspoiled haven, Gauguin set out to embody them in his life and work. A prosperous stockbroker and avid art collector, whose inventory included works by Daumier, Monet, Renoir, Manet, Cézanne, and Pissarro, he abandoned the Paris business scene and his brood of five children to devote his life to art at age 35. Giving up comfort, commercial success, and artistic acclaim, he embraced isolation to know primitive idyll and find the core truth missing from his life.

He sought solace at first in Brittany among the peasants of the French countryside and then in the far away islands of the South Pacific, whose promise of paradise on earth lured many others, among them, Herman Melville, Mark Twain, and Robert Louis Stevenson. Under the blazing sun of the Polynesian islands, where as he put it in his copious writings, "the material necessities of life can be had without money," Gauguin articulated his artistic sentiment into original work that influenced generations to come. Synthesizing elements of his admired contemporaries, Cézanne, van Gogh, and others, and inspired by Japanese prints, folk art, and medieval stained glass, he created exuberant tableaux charged with sensuality and primal tension.

Gauguin's life as adoptive "savage" was one of unrelenting hardship, for the primitive idyll existed only in his inflamed imagination. From the moment he arrived on the islands, he was plagued by two of the many motivators of civilization, poverty and disease. Unable to afford even painting supplies and weakened by malnutrition and syphilis, he moved from Martinique to Tahiti and finally the Marquesas Islands, where he died at age 53.

Gauguin's art expressed his vision of the world. The edge of the canvas did not frame the images but rather opened them to wider exploration. Unspoiled nature was bountiful and generous, warm, forgiving, and open. Like his paintings, it had no boundaries, and its essence existed only in the imagination. Even as his body failed and his resources expired, its lure did not fray, nor did his zeal for it diminish.

Unlike civilized society, whose joyless monotone had alienated him, the primitive idyll had not been meddled with or manipulated. Unregulated and unrestrained, it followed nature's rhythm. Painted in startling, unnatural colors that punctuated the spiritual as well as the physical, it had a languid but steady beat. In the moist heat, laboriously outlined flat figures of humans and animals shared a communal living, even if it was not, as Gauguin wished it, altogether loving and harmless.

The prickly pandanus (screw pine), whose symbolic abundance pervades the namesake painting, is native to many Pacific archipelagoes, providing roof, sustenance, adornment, and medicine to generations of islanders. Filtering the sea breezes and moderating the tropical heat, the pandanus shelters the underbrush, which contains the complex ecosystem at the heart of the tropics' languid beat.

Undergrowth vegetation in tropical and subtropical areas is home to countless creatures (mammals, reptiles, birds) that sustain sandflies, ticks, fleas, and mosquitoes, whose complex natural cycles flourish in the heat and humidity so central to Gauguin's Eden. Unnoticed and unpainted, these vectors nurture the dark underpinning of untamed nature, including arthropod-borne diseases: sleeping sickness in Uganda; dengue in Cuba, French Guiana, Bangladesh, and Myanmar; cutaneous leishmaniasis in Colombia; malaria in Western Kenya; West Nile virus in Guadeloupe; murine virus in the Canary Islands.

Bibliography

Gauguin P. *Noa, Noa: The Tahiti Journal of Paul Gauguin.* California, CA: Chronicle Books; 1994.

The Great Masters. London, England: Quantum Publishing; 2003.

Pandanus tectorius. Available at: http://www.comfsm.fm/~dleeling/angio/pandanus.html. Accessed April 25, 2013.

Vol.11, No.10, October 2005

DEPARTMENT OF
HEALTH & HUMAN SERVICES
Public Health Service
Centers for Disease Control and Prevention (CDC)
Atlanta, GA 30333

Official Business
Penalty for Private Use $300

Return Service Requested

MEDIA MAIL
POSTAGE & FEES PAID
PHS/CDC
Permit No. G-284

EMERGING INFECTIOUS DISEASES

A Peer-Reviewed Journal Tracking and Analyzing Disease Trends   Vol.11, No.10, October 2005

EID Online
www.cdc.gov/eid

Water-related Illness

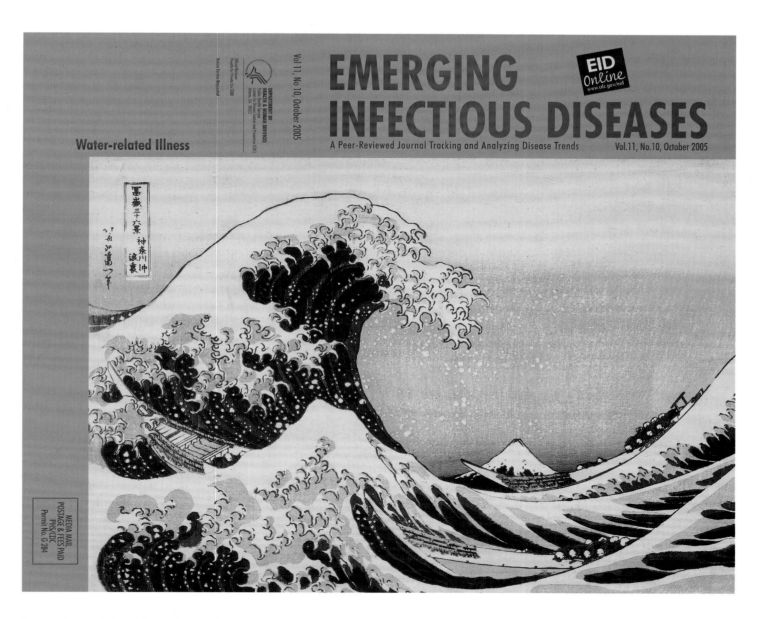

富嶽三十六景 神奈川沖 浪裏

Emerg. Infect. Dis., Vol. 11, No. 10, Oct. 2005

OF TIDAL WAVES AND HUMAN FRAILTY

"From the age of 6, I had a penchant for copying the form of things, and from about 50, my pictures were frequently published; but until the age of 70, nothing that I drew was worthy of notice," wrote Katsushika Hokusai in his autobiography. "At 73 years, I was somewhat able to fathom the growth of plants and trees; and the structure of birds, animals, insects and fish. Thus when I reached 80 years, I hope to have made increasing progress, and at 90 to see further into the underlying principles of things, so that at 100 years I will have achieved a divine state in my art, and at 110, every dot and every stroke will be as though alive."

"The old man mad about painting" was how Hokusai signed some of his work. Passion for art defined his life. And on his deathbed, at age 89, he bemoaned, "If only Heaven will give me just another 10 years . . . just another 5 more years, then I could become a real painter."

Hokusai was born in Edo, present-day Tokyo. He showed early interest in art and was apprenticed to Katsukawa Shunsho, master painter and printmaker, to paint *ukiyo-e*, "images of the floating world," a style focused on everyday activities and their fleeting nature. He painted the transient lives of actors in Edo's theater district, then moved on to study other art styles and become famous for his illustrations of poetry and popular novels. He drew from diverse artistic traditions, among them Chinese and Western art, which was then beginning to appear in Japan. Versatile and prolific, he left thousands of works, signed in more than 30 artistic names. He created a series of sketchbooks as instruction to those who wanted to draw in his style. The series was called Hokusai manga, a term he coined.

In a traditional society of Confucian values and rigid regimentation, Hokusai was bohemian. Eccentric, rebellious, and temperamental, he cared nothing about convention and was reputed to move each time the notorious clutter and disorder of his home became unbearable. Legend has it that when invited once to paint maple leaves floating on the Tatsuta River, he drew a few blue lines and then repeatedly imprinted atop the scroll chicken's feet he had dipped into red color. When his contemporaries drew the shoguns and samurai, he portrayed the common people, and when he painted landscapes, it was strictly from his own point of view.

Even though Hokusai's work did not receive full appreciation in Japan, it gained high status and respect abroad. *The Great Wave* became a global icon, as recognizable and revered as Leonardo da Vinci's *Mona Lisa* or Vincent van Gogh's *Sunflowers*. Hokusai prints were collected by Claude Monet, Edgar Degas, Mary Cassatt, and many others, who were influenced by them.

Hokusai reached the peak of his creativity in his 70s, when he began work on his *Thirty-six views of Mount Fuji* (3,776 m), Japan's summit and spiritual epicenter. These images, like much of his mature work, reflect familiarity with such European trends as innovative pigments and the telescope. Fascinated by

Western design principles, he integrated them with Japanese technique, not only in landscape paintings but also with flowers and birds, which he showed in horizontal close-ups and cutouts as if seen by a telescope. His imaginative efforts captured the essence rather than the likeness of what he painted and created an altogether novel effect, which appeared Japanese to outsiders and Western to the Japanese.

The Great Wave is Hokusai's most celebrated work. Although renowned nature scenes featured often in Japanese art, the landscape as *ukiyo-e* theme did not gain prominence until after views of Mount Fuji prints became popular. *The Great Wave* inspired other artistic works, as diverse as Rainer Maria Rilke's poem "Der Berg" ("The Mountain") and Claude Debussy's symphonic masterpiece *La Mer* (The Sea), whose full score featured *The Great Wave* on its first edition at the request of the composer.

This refined woodblock print epitomizes the artist's skills. Although meticulously structured, it appears effortless, its flair equaled only by the purity of its composition. Undulating lines are fine, at times almost invisible, the colors deliberate and intense. The viewer is guided through the perilous ebb, past the boats to the landmark mountain. The wave is menacing and ghostly, hardened by thick skeletal lines, softened by bubbles of mist, sparkling and voluminous. An eerie feeling is punctuated by the pale sky and frosty white of breaking waves and mountain peak.

The scene could not be more *ukiyo-e*: three light boats carrying fish to market on a work day. But on this day, the sea is in charge, a monstrous wave commanding the foreground, cresting high above the horizon, dwarfing majestic Mt. Fuji now a bump in the fluid scene. Like leaves tossed to sea, the boats tumble, their tiny occupants crouched in fear, clinging to the sides, unable to face the wave and its claws of foam curling toward them.

In *The Great Wave*, Hokusai captured the uneasy sentiments of a nation surrounded and defined by water, as well as the deeper, primal, human terror of the sea. Enchanting but treacherous, water lures and repels. Seeking livelihood, fortune, adventure, or just solace in its calm, humans ride the waves, risking capricious tempests, settling in precarious coastal regions frequently battered and overpowered by the sea. When the earth moves or climate and other elements stir the waters, environmental markers shift, boats and settlements crumble, and humans perish. In the aftermath comes infectious disease, originating in the disruption and lingering for lack of hygienic conditions and adequate medical care.

Hokusai's fishermen typify human plight against overwhelming force. Their posture embodies the horror of imminent physical harm and death. Fear and anxiety about the long-term consequences of environmental catastrophe are left to survivors and public health workers, who face, along with the loss of infrastructure, compromised sanitation, contamination of water supplies, secondary wound infections, unsafe food, increased poverty, and compounded disease.

The formidable challenge of water-related illness and death persists, from the Indian Ocean to the Gulf of Mexico—despite global prevention and control efforts. Like the fishermen caught in Hokusai's wave, unable to confront the culprit, we cling to a lifeline: managing the physical trauma and addressing resultant infections and complications.

Bibliography

Hokusai FM. *Mountains and Water, Flowers and Birds*. Munich, Germany: Prestel; 2004.

Impressionist influences in the music of Claude Debussy. Available at: http://www.tcd.ie/Music/JF%20History/debussy.html. Accessed April 25, 2013.

Kita S, Kobayashi T. The bohemian vs. the bureaucrat: Hokusai and Hiroshige. Available at: http://www.carnegiemuseums.org/cmag/bk_issue/1996/marapr/hokusai.htm. Accessed April 25, 2013.

Vol 11, No 11, November 2005

EMERGING
INFECTIOUS DISEASES

A Peer-Reviewed Journal Tracking and Analyzing Disease Trends

Vol.9, No.4, April 2003

EID
Online
www.cdc.gov/eid

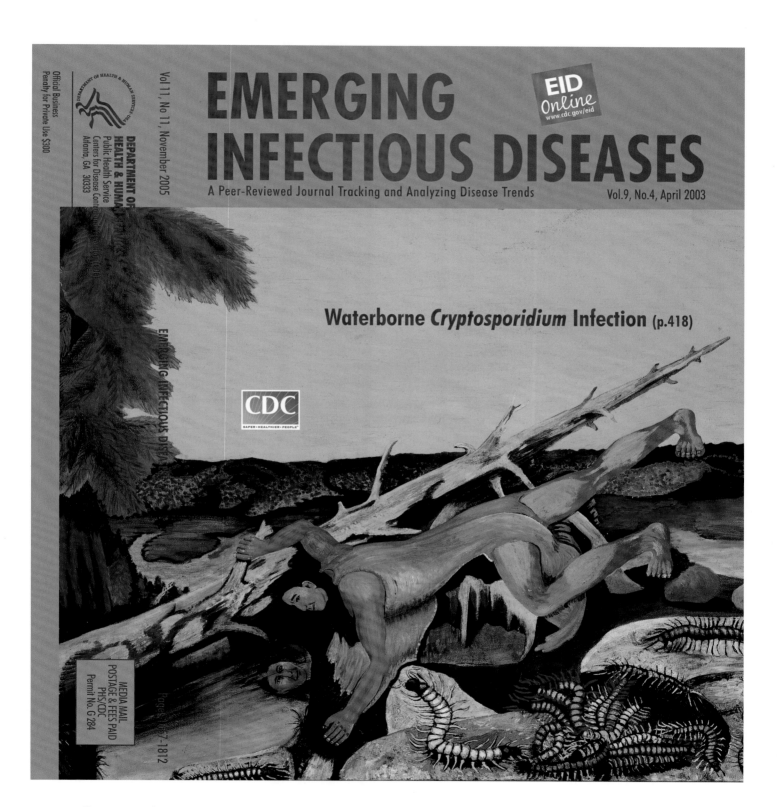

Waterborne *Cryptosporidium* Infection (p.418)

CDC
SAFER · HEALTHIER · PEOPLE

MEMORY AND IMAGINATION AS PREDICTORS OF HARM

"Once in while I take up color and paint a little bit because if I do not do this, all things will be forgotten," Frank Day said of his work. The artist, who was born into the Konkow Maidu tribe in Berry Creek, California, was also a gifted storyteller and teacher as well as talented artist, Day translated this tribal perception of the world into narrative images filled with Maidu themes in bold color.

Like many Native Americans of his generation, Day was under pressure throughout his life to abandon Native cultural practices in the interest of assimilation. A boarding-school student, he grew up wearing a standard school uniform and learning the ways of the broader society. But after the death of his father in 1922, Day set off to explore the history, language, ceremonies, and customs he had learned from him and other tribal elders. For a decade, he traveled western areas that had been inhabited by Indian tribes for hundreds of years and finally settled in California, where he worked as an agricultural laborer. After a serious injury, he turned to art as therapy. Without formal training, he soon exhibited untapped artistic talent and pure, distinctive style.

In the more than 200 canvasses he painted in the last two decades of his life, Day integrated myth, legend, and oral tradition into powerful compositions. His paintings, created from memory rather than observation, had a dreamy, symbolic, and imaginative bend. Rough brushstrokes, rich texture, and raw emotive color invoked the spiritual underpinnings of cultural traditions rather than the traditions themselves. The paintings contained strong intuitive structure and contemporary elegance.

Day's "cultural memory" refuted presumptions that the California Indians were vanishing, and he was heralded for his inspiring presence during the revitalization of California Indian arts in the 1960s and 1970s. His artistic contributions were celebrated in "Memory and Imagination," a major exhibit organized by the Oakland Museum of California in 1997. Day's works are an authoritative tribute to Native American heritage and its focus on the spiritual connection between humanity and nature.

Infectious diseases, from smallpox and plague to tuberculosis and influenza, featured in many of the Indian legends whose essence Day sought to preserve. Blending the dangerous with the supernatural, these legends weaved historical accounts into tales of mystery, medicine, and magic and celebrated the creative spirit with which Native tribes approached disease survival. One painting, *The Burning of the Roadhouse*, commemorated therapeutic burning of dwellings to rid them of disease; another, *Sunflower Remedy*, portrayed a dazzling sunflower shielding a child from tuberculosis.

The Water Test is a culmination of Day's Native Indian and artistic philosophy: everything is interconnected and imbued with spiritual energy that can be positive or negative. In this symbolic composition, human presence is in center stage. The pastoral scene, afloat in nature, is spare and horizontal but full of vitality. Water, a critical element providing not only physical but also spiritual sustenance, is set off by dramatic earth tones, balanced on the left by a thriving tree and in the diagonal center by a fallen one, which (as if charged by unknown energy) stretches to infinity.

A man leans over the water, perhaps to test whether it is clear enough to drink or warm enough to get into. Distracted by his reflection, he assumes a narcissistic posture and smiles at his robust image, his own character now being playfully tested by the water. His body is perfectly balanced and in control, but his relationship with the environment seems ambiguous. The water bank is teeming with oversized centipedes, some lurking in bellicose conference under a rock, some venturing out for prey. Their proximity, inflammatory colors, and poised poisoned fangs exude hostility.

The realistic encounter of man and water is embroidered with fantasy. The water contains invisible seeds of harm. The artist, acknowledging that the man's water test is as vain and elusive as his reflected image, pulls out of the water and into the foreground the centipedes, crude indicators of harm amplified and exposed to the naked eye.

Our water tests are more refined now, but they still seek indicators of harm. While we search for better evidence of their presence, harmful critters remain hidden. Standard plate counts or coliform counts are reasonable predictors of microbial presence, but as we peer deeply into our water, other microbes—noroviruses, Giardia, Cryptosporidium—continue to elude us, testing our essential drinking water and our survival.

Bibliography

McFarlan AA, ed. *American Indian Legends.* New York, NY: Heritage Press; 1968.

Walkingstick K, Marshall AE. *So Fine! Masterworks of Fine Art from the Heard Museum.* Phoenix, AZ: Heard Museum; 2001.

Wasserman A. Memory and imagination: the legacy of Maidu Indian artist Frank Day; http://www.museumca.org/exhibit/exhi_memory_imagination.html; accessed February 19, 2003.

Wilson DB. Frank Day: memories and imagination. Available at: http://www.nativepeoples.com/Native-Peoples/January-February-1998/Frank-Day-Memories-and-Imagination/. Accessed April 27, 2013.

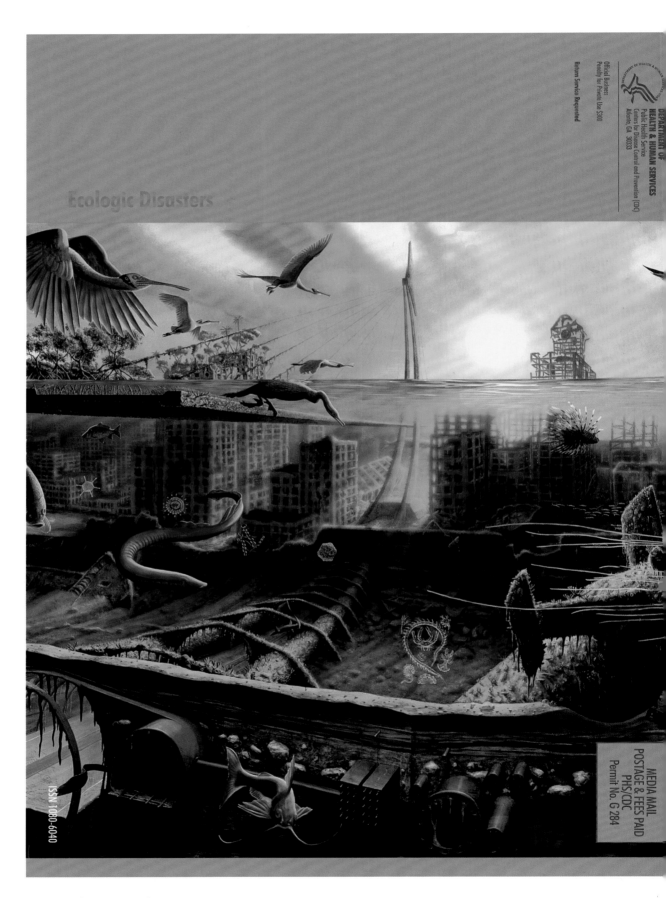

Ecologic Disasters

ISSN 1080-6040

EMERGING INFECTIOUS DISEASES®

EID Online
www.cdc.gov/eid

April 2006

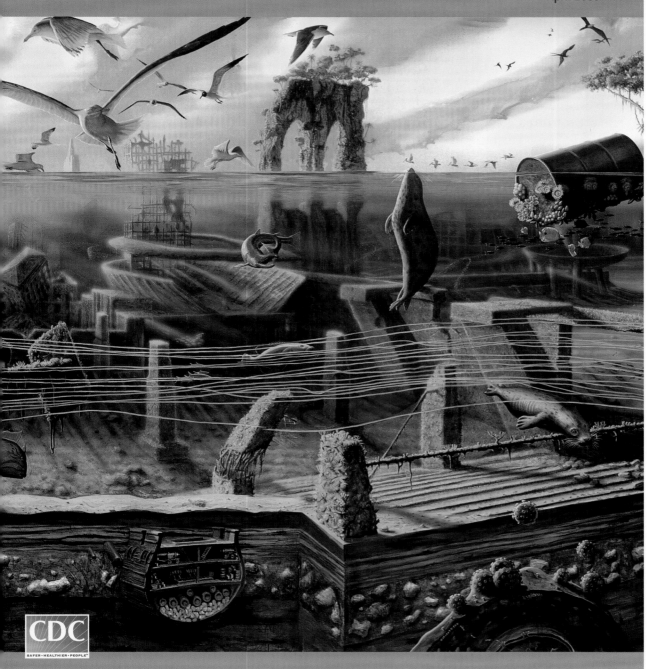

CDC
SAFER · HEALTHIER · PEOPLE™

MANIFESTING ECOLOGIC AND MICROBIAL CONNECTIONS

"I'm a pop artist using natural history as my iconography," Alexis Rockman has said of himself. Pop art, a movement that coincided with the youth and music phenomena of the 1950s and 1960s, draws its subject matter from the modern urban consumer experience, adopting popular culture icons and introducing them to the art world, much as American artist Andy Warhol incorporated and immortalized in his work canned soup and actress Marilyn Monroe. A man of his times, Rockman lives and breathes the culture of his native New York City, drawing inspiration from it, absorbing its trends, obsessions, conflicts, and fears, which he then brings to life in fantastic images created from nature.

Apart from a brief stay in a remote area of Peru, where his mother, anthropologist Diana Wall, did field work, Rockman grew up an urban child in an Upper East Side apartment oddly populated with newts, cats, boa constrictors, iguanas, tortoises, and lizards. He collected specimens and kept poisonous dart frogs, which he drew from a very young age, and planned to be a scientist. His playground was the American Museum of Natural History, where his mother worked with anthropologist Margaret Mead. The museum's extensive collections and dioramas became an influential part of his childhood. The artists who created the dioramas, he later said, were guided by the same painters who inspired him, Thomas Cole, Frederic Church, Albert Bierstadt.

His interest in zoology and botany was rivaled by other interests, among them film making and animation. He studied at the Rhode Island School of Design and graduated from New York's School of Visual Arts with a major in illustration. He worked as columnist and illustrator for *Natural History* magazine, while he gradually moved toward fine arts and started to show his work in solo and group exhibitions. A major influence was artist Ross Bleckner, whom he served as assistant for a time and who advised him to move toward modernism.

A leader among contemporary artists returning to figurative content, Rockman wants to paint what he sees. Taken with the natural world, he studies not only nature's creatures but also the puzzles surrounding them: their origins, survival, adaptability, and evolution. Plants and animals are photographed and researched in libraries, their native habitats, or the Bronx Zoo. He delves into taxonomy and molecular biology and has enlisted the help and gained the following of paleontologists, biologists, ecologists, ichthyologists, and other scientists, who provide him clues to the accuracy of his exacting images. He has traveled to the rainforests of Brazil and Guyana in search of authentic specimens and to the South Pacific to sketch the extinct Tasmanian tiger in a local laboratory. He counts Charles Darwin as a mentor.

A combination of natural science and fantasy, his work explores the predatory relationship between nature and culture. Inspired equally by scientific curiosity and artistic compulsion, his startling images are at once literal, naturalistic, and entirely imaginary. Challenging the way we see and categorize the world, he questions human–animal nature interaction by creating "in your face" scenarios based on vital popular culture dilemmas, among them genetic engineering and global warming.

"He tweaks my cerebrum," late professor Stephen Jay Gould said of Rockman. His snakes grow legs and chickens sport multiple sets of wings. Kangaroo-sized rats stroll across futuristic landscapes. A pig harbors human organs for harvest, and grossly oversized parasites, ticks, ants, and viruses populate his large surreal scenes. Botanical compositions, swarming with nature's less appreciated creatures and extinct or mutant forms feature aquatic or tree-sized dandelions. Humans are rarely present, though human handiwork always is. Riddles and humor are mixed in with actual soil, mud, sand, vegetation, and other collage materials, adding tactile interest to rich layers of color and varnish, which create a highly finished, luminous effect.

For nearly two decades, Rockman has worked from his studio in TriBeCa, transforming historical culture into naturalistic images. Referring to himself as a "paleo-geek," he favors large prehistoric landscapes reinterpreting the ecologic past and still lifes exploring the evolutionary future.

In *Manifest Destiny*, Rockman imagines Brooklyn 3,000 years in the future. Fueled by exhaustive research, his artistic imagination produces a panoramic view of Brooklyn Bridge and environs. The polar ice caps have melted and the borough is under water. An eerie orange glow permeates layers of underwater ruins covered with slime and inhabited by weird creatures. In what the painter has referred to as "democratic space," prehistoric beasts paddle with newfangled mutants and every-day pests.

"I'm dying to see what scientists will think," Rockman said, while still working on the painting, transforming technical information from his research into visual language. In this restructured environment, geology is turned on its ear, along with the food chain. Large fish with snake heads or oversized whiskers swim by a tire-like cell infected with giant HIV. Jellyfish tentacles stretch halfway across the sea-scape, past a two-tailed salmon. Flocks of wild birds hover above the waterline. Minute life forms, enlarged against the ruins, signal the survival of the unexpected. A galleon rests near the wreckage of a nuclear submarine. And the grand bridge lies broken, a fossil amidst decaying structures and vegetation.

Rockman's haunting vision of the future is rife with cultural and evolutionary undertones. The geologic, botanical, and zoologic clues to the future, rooted in the past and buried in the lurid reds of rust and pollution, are well understood by scientists. For ecologic disaster and disease emergence evolve along the same path, guided by the same factors: human demographics and behavior, technology and industry, economic development and land use, international travel and commerce, microbial adaptation and change, and the breakdown of public health measures.

And while short-term risk for epidemics after geophysical disasters may be low, long-term effects of ecologic change on disease emergence, aptly shown in the exaggerated size of viruses (e.g., HIV), are huge. Rockman's meticulously drawn mutants, alluding to genetic engineering or environmental pollution, also articulate dilemmas inherent in disease control: because of microbes' evolutionary potential, our very drugs or pesticides may contribute to selection of mutations, adaptations, and migrations that enable pathogens to proliferate and nonpathogens to become virulent. Manifest or not, the destiny of humans, animals, and the natural environment is inextricably interlinked.

Bibliography

Floret N, Viel J-F, Mauny F, et al. Negligible risk for epidemics after geophysical disasters. *Emerg Infect Dis*. 2006;12:543–548.

Gould SJ, Crary J, Quammen D. *Alexis Rockman*. New York, NY: Monacelli Press; 2004.

Mittelbach M, Crewdson M. *Carnivorous Nights: On The Trail of the Tasmanian Tiger*. New York, NY: Villard Books; 2005.

Yablonsky L. New York's watery new grave. *The New York Times*. April 11, 2004;Section 2:28.

Economic Development and Land Use

Economic development can have unintended impact on the environment by causing ecologic changes that alter the replication and transmission patterns of pathogens. Dam building, for example, changes the environment in which pathogens, disease carriers, and host animals coexist because it involves clearing, excavation, and flooding of large areas of land. Construction of the Three Gorges Dam across the Yangtze River will substantially change the ecology of the Dongting Lake in southern China. Among the many effects of the dam will be the likely extension of snail habitats and increase in schistosome transmission and cases of schistosomiasis, a parasitic disease that especially affects children who swim or play in contaminated water. The socioeconomic effects of schistosomiasis are second only to those of malaria. Thomas Eakins's *John Biglin in a Single Scull*, one of the covers in this chapter, ties economic development, a factor in emergence, with deterioration of water quality and its public health consequences.

Deforestation and subsequent reforestation can have similar effects. Albrecht Dürer's *Stag Beetle* focuses on a humble creature now endangered along with many others as its woodsy habitat disappears. In the early 1800s, the eastern United States became virtually treeless when large tracts of land were cleared for agriculture. As forests disappeared, the deer population decreased. In the mid-1800s, US agriculture moved westward to the Great Plains. Abandoned farms soon were retaken by forests in large portions of the East. Unlike primeval forest, this new woodland was choked with undergrowth and contained no predators large enough to regulate deer populations. The deer proliferated, and later, people began to cohabitate forested areas with the wildlife. The proximity of humans, mice, deer, and ticks was an ideal opening for the Lyme disease spirochete, which is spread by the bite of certain ticks. Lyme disease is now the most common vectorborne infection in the United States.

Urbanization also affects the reemergence of disease. Daudi E. S. Tingatinga's *Leopard*, a colorful cover in this chapter, touches on some of the risks posed by expansion of human communities into the wild on all continents, including Africa. Road building has opened up opportunities for bushmeat hunting, which increased hunters' risk for exposure to infection during handling, rendering, and transporting game. Increased consumption of bushmeat may have been instrumental in the early emergence of HIV.

As human development encroaches on the forest and transforms the native environment, mosquitoes travel to new areas. These adaptable insects have become domesticated, anthropophilic, and therefore dangerous to humans. Changes in the behavior of mosquitoes fuel the reemergence of tropical infections like dengue, with millions of cases each year and thousands of deaths. Dengue fever, once restricted to poor people in tropical areas, is now an equal opportunity disease, threatening affluent urbanites and poor inner-city residents alike. Eugene von Guérard's *Ferntree Gully in the Dandenong Ranges* shows unspoiled wilderness before human development could interfere with nature's cycles, promoting the reemergence of tropical disease.

Integrated pig-duck agriculture, an extremely efficient food production system practiced in certain parts of China for centuries, may be the origin of pandemic influenza, whose viruses have generally come from Asia. Pandemic influenza viruses, unlike strains that cause annual or biennial epidemics, do not generally result from mutation of viruses circulating in humans. Instead, they result from reassortment. Gene segments from two influenza strains, at least one of which has not caused human infections, produce a new virus with surface characteristics different from those of virus strains that have been infecting humans. Waterfowl are major reservoirs of influenza viruses, and pigs can serve as mixing vessels where avian and swine viruses can trade genes and produce new mammalian influenza strains.

Integrated farming puts two species, swine and birds, in contact and provides a natural laboratory for new influenza recombinants. Close contact of ducks, pigs, and people; international trade in potentially infected animals; and global travel all contribute to the development and spread of the next pandemic influenza virus. With high-intensity agriculture and movement of livestock across borders, suitable conditions may also arise in Europe. *Phoenix and Birds*, a silk scroll from China and a cover in this chapter, offers a composite image, the Chinese version of the phoenix, a fitting metaphor for the wild recombinations of the flu virus and the potential for emergence of a new virus with pandemic potential.

Environmental changes bring people and their domestic animals into closer contact with wildlife hosts of pathogens. Up to 75% of human emerging infectious diseases are caused by zoonotic pathogens, that is, infectious agents that can be transmitted between or are shared by animals and humans. These include pathogens responsible for massive deaths around the globe (HIV, influenza virus) and others that cause few deaths but for which no effective therapies or vaccines exist (Ebola virus, Nipah virus, SARS coronavirus). *The Painted Gallery Ceiling, Lascaux Caves* reminds of the complex relationship between animals and humans, a relationship that started millions of years ago. George Seurat's *Sunday Afternoon on the Island of La Grande Jatte*, because of its pointillist style, invites a connection between the painting and the viewer, whose eyes must connect the points to see the image. Other connections, unintended by the artist, can also be made, such as the unseen biological one between the strolling crowd, their pets, and the microbes they share.

Bibliography

Hwang SW, Svoboda TJ, De Jong IJ, et al. Bed bug infestations in an urban environment. *Emerg Infect Dis.* 2005;1111:533–538.

Nesje P. Tingatinga art in Tanzania: the predicament of culture? *Postamble.* 2004;1(1); 2004.

Potter P. Fearsome creatures and nature's gothic. Available at: http://wwwnc.cdc.gov/eid/article/11/4/ac-1104_article.htm. Accessed June 4, 2013.

Potter P. He who dines with the leopard is liable to be eaten. Available at: http://wwwnc.cdc.gov/eid/article/12/9/ac-1209_article.htm. Accessed May 11, 2013.

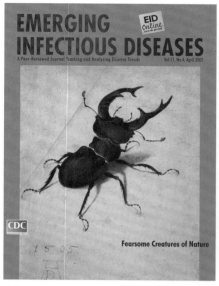

Fearsome Creatures of Nature; http://dx.doi.org/10.3201/eid1104.AC1104

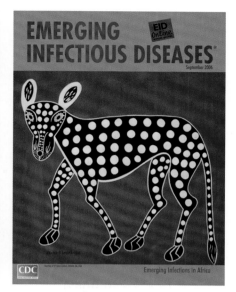

Emerging Infections in Africa; http://dx.doi.org/10.3201/eid1209.AC1209

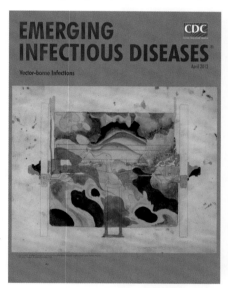

Vector-borne Infections; http://dx.doi.org/10.3201/eid1804.AC1804

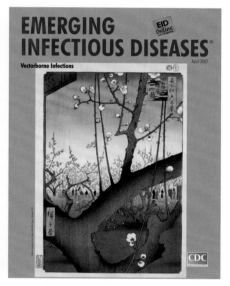

Vector-borne Infections; http://dx.doi.org/10.3201/eid1304.AC1304

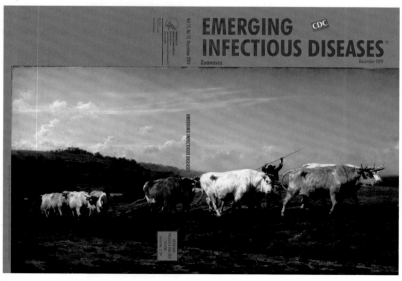

Zoonoses; http://dx.doi.org/10.3201/eid1512.AC1512

EMERGING
INFECTIOUS DISEASES®

July 2007

EID Online
www.cdc.gov/eid

Water-related Illness

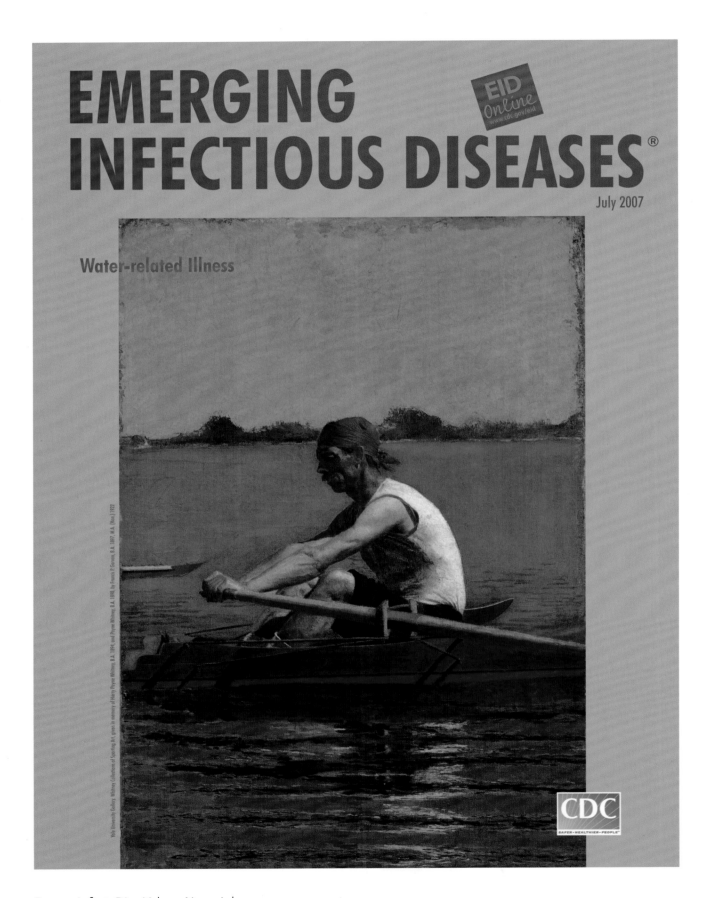

Yale University Gallery. Whitney Collection of Sporting Art, given in memory of Harry Payne Whitney, B.A. 1894, and Payne Whitney, B.A. 1898, by Francis P. Garvan, B.A. 1897, M.A. (Hon.) 1922

CDC
SAFER·HEALTHIER·PEOPLE™

Emerg. Infect. Dis., Vol. 13, No. 7, Jul. 2007

ROWING ON THE SCHUYLKILL, DAMMING ON THE YANGTZE

"Should the he-painters draw the horses and bulls, and the she-painters . . . the mares and cows?" asked Thomas Eakins, when critics derided his use of nude models in the presence of women art students. Eakins made no bones about his teaching practices and no compromises in his pursuit of artistic excellence. So he was viewed as radical and irascible, and although his art was widely discussed and exhibited, he did not see commercial success during his lifetime—he only sold 30 paintings.

A man ahead of his time, Eakins was born in Philadelphia, the son of a calligrapher, who nurtured his artistic talent and taught him the value of exacting detail. "I was born July 25, 1844. My father's father was from the north of Ireland of the Scotch Irish. On my mother's side my blood is English and Hollandish. I was a pupil of Gérôme (also of [portrait painter] Bonnat and Dumont, [the] sculptor). I have taught in life classes and lectured on anatomy continuously since 1873. I have painted many pictures and done a little sculpture. . . . I believe my life is all in my work," he wrote.

Eakins studied drawing at the Pennsylvania Academy of Fine Arts and anatomy at Jefferson Medical College, traveled to Paris to attend the École des Beaux-Arts, and near the end of his studies, visited Spain "to see the pictures." Despite his studies in Paris, he was most influenced by 17th-century Dutch and Spanish painters, particularly Diego Velázquez and Jusepe de Ribera. He lived the rest of his life in his beloved Philadelphia, following his own advice on achieving greatness: "remain in America to peer deeper into the heart of American life."

Philadelphia and the Schuylkill River, which runs through it, held a special fascination for Eakins. He delighted in sailing, swimming, rowing, and all manner of outdoor activity before and after his travels abroad. Rowing, already a popular sport, attracted large crowds in the 1850s, when several rowing clubs formed the Schuylkill Navy, now the oldest amateur athletic governing body in the United States. As Eakins began his career and sought subjects from his immediate surroundings, he got caught up in the excitement of the sport, becoming one of the first artists to portray rowers in action. Sometimes he placed himself in the pictures and inscribed his name on the scull.

His painting of the human form, encouraged during his studies from nude models in Paris, was all but stifled by local culture, but the seminude athletic figure was socially acceptable. He produced nearly 30 rowing pictures from 1871 to 1874, at first painting his childhood friend Max Schmitt and later the Biglin brothers, a pair of celebrity rowers from New York. Still, reviews in the *Philadelphia Inquirer* were not glowing: "The artist, in dealing so boldly and broadly with the commonplace in nature, is working upon well-supported theories, and, despite somewhat scattered effect, gives promise of a conspicuous future."

As teacher and later director of the Pennsylvania Academy of the Fine Arts, he introduced anatomy, dissection, and scientific perspective into the curriculum, revolutionizing art instruction. But he also scandalized school authorities with the use of nude models and was forced to resign in 1886. He continued to paint. "I will never have to give up painting, for even now I could paint heads good enough to make a living anywhere in America." Later he was recognized for his formidable talent and was elected to the National Academy of Design. Provocative behavior, however, continued to damage his reputation: "My honors are misunderstanding, persecution, and neglect."

Eakins's approach to painting relied on close observation. He rejected embellishment and sentimentality and was the only artist, his friend Walt Whitman said, "who could resist the temptation to see what [he] think[s] ought to be rather than what is." During the latter part of his career, he focused on portraiture: studies of relatives, friends, and persons accomplished in the sciences and other disciplines. The subject of a fine portrait in 1888, Whitman called Eakins "not so much a painter, as a force." Unlike his contemporaries James McNeill Whistler, John Singer Sargent, and William Merritt Chase, popular society portraitists, Eakins painted his subjects with uncompromising realism and meticulous precision, which lent them a somber, aged, sometimes unflattering, aspect. While Chase's studio was an atelier, Eakins joked, his own was a workshop.

One of his portraits, *The Gross Clinic*, widely acclaimed as the greatest American painting of the 19th century, depicts surgeon Samuel D. Gross performing surgery, instructing students, and training assistants to remove bone from the leg of an anesthetized patient. The portrait scandalized Victorian society. "It is a picture that even strong men find it difficult to look at long, if they can look at it at all"; wrote *The New York Tribune*, "and as for people with nerves and stomachs, the scene is so real that they might as well go to a dissecting room and have done with it."

In *John Biglin in a Single Scull*, Eakins brought to bear his personal experience as rower and knowledge of the muscles involved. John Biglin, a "physical specimen . . . about as near perfect as can be found," dominated the rowing scene in the 1860s and 1870s. Sculpted as in relief, the figure is focused and intense, muscles terse, shoulders rounded. The composition is economical and accurate, from the sports hero's facial features to the slightly worn wooden thole pin that held the oar in place for rowing. John Biglin, the quintessential outdoorsman equivalent of Samuel Gross the heroic physician!

Water activities continue on the Schuylkill and elsewhere, and the excitement of rowing remains undiminished as does the enjoyment of art. Our close relationship with water, far more complex than Eakins's luminous river would suggest, has only become closer with better understanding of biology. In the 1850s, while rowing was becoming popular in Philadelphia, John Snow, the "father of epidemiology," was investigating the water supply and sewage disposal in South London and finding that cholera is waterborne.

More than a hundred years later, diarrhea is the leading cause of childhood deaths in places that must rely on drinking water contaminated with pathogens. Invasive water organisms are spreading fast around the globe, damaging agriculture. And human activities, such as the Three Gorges Dam construction across the Yangtze River in the People's Republic of China, are threatening changes in ecology and setbacks in schistosomiasis control.

Water quality has environmental and social components. It is like good painting, which Eakins believed, extends beyond the geometry of landscape and the refraction of light on the waves to provide full understanding. Or, as he put it, "You can see what o'clock it is afternoon or morning if it's hot or cold winter or summer and what kind of people are there and what they are doing and why they are doing it."

Bibliography

Li Y-S, Faso G, Zhao Z-Y, et al. Large water management projects and schistosomiasis control, Dongting Lake Region, China. *Emerg Infect Dis.* 2007;13:973–979.

Sewell D. *Thomas Eakins: Artist of Philadelphia.* Philadelphia, PA: Philadelphia Museum of Art; 1982.

Stockman LJ, Fischer TK, Deming M, et al. Point-of-use water treatment and use among mothers in Malawi. *Emerg Infect Dis.* 2007;13:1077–1080.

Wang Q-P, Chen X-G, Lun Z-R. Invasive fresh water snail, China [letter]. *Emerg Infect Dis.* 2007;13:1119–1120.

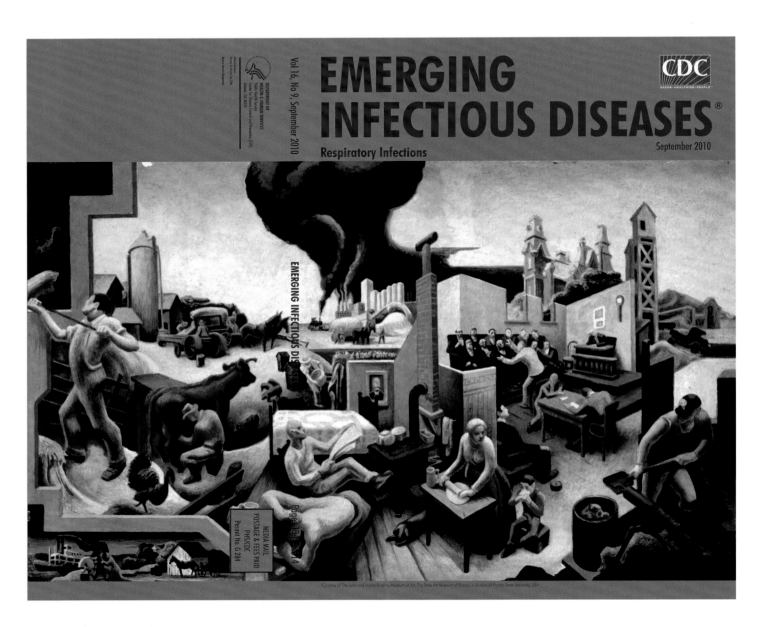

THE SOOT THAT FALLS FROM CHIMNEYS

"The best damned painter in America" is how Harry S. Truman described Thomas Hart Benton, his choice to create a mural for the Truman Library in Independence, Missouri. The President's fellow Missourian lived in Kansas City at the time, his artistic career in a slump, though his reputation as a fine muralist still intact. "I picked him," Mr. Truman told the crowd at the mural's dedication, "because he was the best, and this is the finest work by the best."

During work on the Library mural, the President noted that he got along with the painter, even though, he joked, "That's hard for anyone to do." A gifted musician, writer, and prolific lithographer, Benton was also direct, impatient, radical, and often tactless. He hated museums, professing that artworks belonged in clubs and barrooms, "Anywhere anybody had time to look at 'em." In his autobiography, he mused, "A few people have, at times, expressed a belief that I was not the most desirable kind of fellow to have around. But, all in all, my differences with the home folks, when looked at in perspective, have not amounted to much."

Born in a fiercely political family, the artist was named after his uncle Thomas Hart Benton, the first and longest serving US Senator of Missouri. His father, a populist, was a member of the US House of Representatives. Benton bucked family tradition and entered the Art Institute of Chicago, in 1907, aspiring to become a cartoonist. His longtime love of painting affirmed in the fine arts environment, he traveled to Paris, where he attended the Académie Julien and Académie Colarossi. He met Mexican muralist Diego Rivera and studied the masters at the Louvre, among them El Greco, whose exaggerated forms found their way into his mature style.

Back in New York for the lack of funds, he explored the local scene and such prevailing styles as impressionism and synchromism, especially in the work of Stanton MacDonald-Wright, who became his friend. His career took a different turn when he joined the Navy. "The most important thing, so far, I had ever done for myself as an artist." This work, which involved extensive documentary drafts and drawing, had an enduring effect on his style. "When I came out of the Navy after the First World War, I made up my mind that I wasn't going to be just a studio painter, a pattern maker in the fashion then dominating the art world—as it still does. I began to think of returning to the painting of subjects, subjects with meanings, which people in general might be interested in."

Though by this time well versed in modernism, Benton turned against it unable to embrace its "colored cubes and classic attenuations," rejecting it as "divorced from the common ways of the day." He moved toward naturalistic and representational work focused on the American scene. He taught at the Art Students League, instructing many who went on to become famous in their own right, not the least of them abstract expressionism icon Jackson Pollock. "Even after I had castigated his innovations and he had replied by saying I had been of value to him only as someone to react against, he kept in personal touch with me."

Benton's style, a blend of modern and academic elements, came to be known as regionalism. Others in this movement were Grant Wood, most famous for his *American Gothic*, and John Steuart Curry, who painted life in his native Kansas.

Many criticized their choice of the local over the cosmopolitan, but the regionalists, particularly Benton, struggled with the notion of an authentic American voice long before New York became an art center. "You just can't think of art in terms of progress," Benton explained in an interview, "It is not progressive. It is just different from age to age. One age gets used to a certain kind of art form and thinks that is better, but the next age will deny that thought and go back to some older form. So I wouldn't compare the animal paintings of the cavemen with those of our times or any other times. . . . We were as good, as artists, when we began our history as we are now—sometimes better."

The 1930s, a decade of unprecedented economic hardship in the United States, witnessed renewed interest in history reflected in all aspects of culture. Murals, among them *The Social History of Missouri* in Jefferson City, which Benton considered his masterpiece, were part of this resurgence, recording as they were milestones in the country's development. Benton captured his era's transformation from rural and agrarian to urban and industrial. He painted the growth of business and technology, and the consequent changes in the lives of the common people, in paintings of steamboats and trains, factories, logging and mining operations, offices and farmhouses. "History was not a scholarly study for me but a drama." He was innovative, bold, outspoken, and unafraid of controversy, allowing myth to blend with observation, casting ordinary people as heroes and pioneers. "I wasn't so much interested in famous characters as I was in Missouri and the ordinary run of Missourians that I'd known in my life."

Benton made a habit of gallivanting around the countryside, meeting people and sketching them and their surroundings. Later he would lay out his designs from these pencil sketches, using pen and ink to define and preserve them. These and three-dimensional clay models he created served as prototypes for oil and tempera studies and for larger compositions. While many critics objected to his subjects, bold colors, manipulated forms, or muscular style, few found fault with his compositional and architectural skills. He had a talent for incorporating multiple themes in limited space and still maintaining cohesiveness.

Interior of a Farmhouse offers a glimpse of the brilliant color, energy, and movement that characterize Benton's art and the complexity and richness of his murals. The title understates this intricate composition. The farmhouse at center stage anchors a community of scenes connected by a fence here, a doorway there, an angle, a partial wall, and contains his favorite people: workers doing what they do in the kitchen, the barn, the fields, at rest. On the periphery, steamboat navigation and the wheels of industry are rolling, their ubiquitous smokestacks belching above the Missouri River. Court is in progress; a worker reads the daily news; another washes up; animals wander in and outdoors. The painter reviews American industry in the 1930s, which pulsates, as if it were a live, breathing organism itself.

The values of honest living and hard labor, at the heart of Benton's work, went hand in hand with the belief that harmony between humans and nature resided on the farm, the interior of which in this painting is not altogether filled with agrarian bliss. Despite the energy emanating from the vibrant community, there are tensions, political and ecologic undertones, part and parcel of industrialization. Benton the social historian sensed the dark side of factories and increased transportation, which he noted in palpable terms, a cloud so menacing against the pristine horizon it unfolded halfway across the painting.

"The yellow smoke that rubs its muzzle on the window-panes / . . . Let fall upon its back the soot that falls from chimneys," Benton's fellow Missourian T. S. Eliot wrote prophetically in "The Love Song of J. Alfred Prufrock." As they settle, the dark plumes from smokestacks, a fixture in the artist's work signaling the machine's intrusion, cause havoc in the farmhouse. "The harmony man had with his environment has broken down," he wrote. "Now men build and operate machines they don't understand and whose inner workings they can't even see."

Choked by industrial and other pollution, we have come to resemble Benton's farmhouse, an organism under stress, because "man doesn't escape his environment." The human lung, at the center of the body's complex internal operations, is also affected by external factors in the environment: pollution, infectious agents, allergens. These factors, along with causing many other local and global adverse effects, complicate and aggravate a host of respiratory problems from rhinovirus infection, influenza, and pneumonia, to pneumococcal disease, tuberculosis, and legionellosis, now found to spread around the community from the water tank of a paving machine. Once again, the farmhouse is threatened by what's lurking in "The yellow fog that rubs its back upon the window-panes."

Bibliography

Benton TH. *An Artist in America*. Columbia, MO: University of Missouri Press; 1983.

Coscollá M, Fenollar J, Escribano I, González-Candelas F. Legionellosis outbreak associated with asphalt paving machine, Spain, 2009. *Emerg Infect Dis*. 2010;16:1381–1387.

Harry S. Truman Library and Museum. Oral history interview with Thomas Hart Benton, April 21, 1964. Available at: http://www.trumanlibrary.org/oralhist//benton.htm. Accessed June 22, 2010.

Oral history interview with Thomas Hart Benton, 1872–1985. July 23–24, 1973. Located at: Archives of American Art, Smithsonian Institution, Washington, DC.

Pells RH. *Radical Visions and American Dreams: Culture and Social Thought in the Depression Years*. New York, NY: Harper and Row; 1973.

Priddy B. *Only the Rivers Are Peaceful: Thomas Hart Benton's Missouri Mural*. Independence, MO: Independence Press; 1989.

EMERGING INFECTIOUS DISEASES®

Vector-borne Infections

May 2011

Emerg. Infect. Dis., Vol. 17, No. 5, May 2011

AND THEREFORE I HAVE SAILED THE SEAS AND COME TO THE HOLY CITY OF BYZANTIUM[1]

"One morning, as Gregor Samsa was waking up from anxious dreams, he discovered that in his bed he had been changed into a monstrous verminous bug," wrote Franz Kafka in *The Metamorphosis*. "He lay on his armor-hard back and saw, as he lifted his head up a little, his brown, arched abdomen divided up into rigid bow-like sections. From this height the blanket, just about ready to slide off completely, could hardly stay in place. His numerous legs, pitifully thin in comparison to the rest of his circumference, flickered helplessly before his eyes."

Kafka's nightmarish tale captures the essence of unexpected uncontrollable life-defining horror, likely caused by Gregor Samsa's inability to cope with societal and family pressures. His predicament, much like any severe disfiguring and disabling illness, would isolate and eventually kill him. Transformative experiences have been the domain of poets and artists alike because artistic sensibility heightens awareness of reality, prompting them to seek a better or more comprehensible alternative. Such seems to be the goal of Stelios Faitakis, who from his native Greece has set out to understand and convey to all a meaningful version of the world around him.

"I was raised in the west suburbs of Athens," recounted Faitakis in a 2007 interview, "a place occupied mostly by the working class." A serious injury during childbirth left him with substantial paralysis of the right arm and, despite extensive surgical and other interventions, it would limit his activities, including painting, to his left arm. "Both my parents were workers in a gold chain factory. . . . They are not what we'd call 'artists,' although when I see my mother creating new designs . . . my artistic nature has some root there. . . . Also my grandfather . . . was a good draftsman. . . . I have painted since childhood."

Overcoming family opposition, Faitakis found his way into the prestigious Academy of Fine Arts in Athens, where he set out on his artistic journey, guided as much by his affinity to mathematics as by Eastern mysticism. Suspicious of authority and large organized institutions, he is self-reliant and openly critical of political oppression. "As long as I can remember, I've been an anarchist." He views art as an inclusive and enlightening agent. His first efforts to reach the public came as graffiti—in the streets of his hometown and later on the walls of the Academy. "Working for the public for me means mostly painting outdoors in the open, in the streets, where everyday people pass to go to their jobs. . . . Athens . . . begs to be painted." His murals have now dotted the globe, from European cities to Miami's Wynwood Art District.

"From the beginning, I chose to paint narrative pictures, like a still from a theatrical play: human characters in some environment doing some action—the simplest scenario possible," with hidden meanings, "as an extra for the more demanding eyes." His heavily populated canvases and murals of common folk at work and play have been likened to the paintings of Pieter Bruegel the Elder; Mexican muralism, a monumental form of wall painting accessible to the masses; Japanese screen painting; and the Cretan School, whose style of icon painting, also seen in the work of El Greco, flourished during the late Middle Ages and peaked after the fall of

---

1 William Butler Yeats, "Sailing to Byzantium."

Constantinople, becoming a major force in Greek painting during the 15th through the 17th centuries.

But what has brought Faitakis into his own is a consistent reference to art forms rooted in the Byzantine tradition. "It would never be possible for me to neglect this element. . . . I paint about Humanity and its relation to itself . . . so my characters flow in a golden world. . . . Simple, ordinary colors coexist with metallic/light reflecting colors. . . . The gold refers to eternity, universal time." The tradition relies on exegesis, "Art should be used as a tool for human beings to . . . grow." In Faitakis's work, monastic settings, precipitous mountains, and hermetic deserts unite with urban scenes, political unrest, and common ailments to seek resolution in unorthodox ways. "Art opens the human being to the use of capabilities that our modern civilization has shrunk, such as intuition and inspiration."

In *Kakerlaken sind die Zukunft*, detailed patterns and elements from psychology, the natural sciences, popular wisdom, and political allegory unite with humor and drama to create aggressive commentary. Perspective is achieved by stacking objects on top of each other. Buildings, decaying cities and surroundings, complex geometric and floral designs, and message ribbons portray, without physical barriers or reference to place and time, the universe. Size denotes importance, so the insect containing the urban scene, placed in full frontal position and regalia, spells an ominous message: vermin can outnumber, outdo, and outlive the human community. Larger than life and wearing a person's head, this all-weather vector feeds on poverty, ignorance, disease, and death.

Frustrated by the state of affairs, the painter abandons the mundane and, like W. B. Yeats, sails to Byzantium—not a destination but an idea. For as the poet says, "the only way for the soul to learn to sing is to study "monuments of its own magnificence." In the vernacular of a bygone culture, he transcends reality to transform obscure troublesome prospects to legible content accessible to all. As the Kafkaesque scenario unfolds, modern inventions move in and out of the stylized landscape—a giant electronic screen; helicopters buzzing like giant insects with petal-like rotors, steam haloes, and landing limbs. A tiny human lurks in a shadowy crevice on the side. Beyond exegesis, this eerie scene invites anagogical interpretation.

Much like a scientist with a microscope, Faitakis amplifies figures and their surroundings to take a closer look at vermin and force the viewer to experience their presence and resilience. But in painting this anthropomorphic insect, he also creates an icon of the ubiquitous vector, which transmits viruses, bacteria, and other pathogens between humans and animals, forming a bridge over spatial, behavioral, and ecologic barriers and promoting the emergence of disease. Yellow fever virus is transmitted from monkeys to humans by mosquitoes; Lyme disease, from rodents to humans by ticks. And though Faitakis's insect contains the city, a vector is not just a vessel. Always evolving as part of the elaborate transmission mechanism, a vector provides the pathogen itself with ways to evolve, creating even more opportunities for disease emergence.

The complexity of human-animal-vector interactions underlying *Kakerlaken sind die Zukunft* adds another dimension to Faitakis's surreal universe. And like the sociopolitical elements, these interactions are staggering and require deeper understanding that may reside "as in the gold mosaic of a wall" at the convergence of human behavior, vector biology, climate, and land use.

Bibliography

Bailey S. Stelios Faitakis: finding divinity in human nature. *Art Papers*. 2010;34:23–25.

Finneran RJ, ed. *The Collected Poems of W.B. Yeats*. New York, NY: Simon and Schuster; 1996.

Re-tile.com. The Breeder: Stelios Faitakis. ". . . to a blessed land of new promise." Available at: http://www.re-title.com/exhibitions/archive_TheBreeder6296.asp. Accessed March 15, 2011.

Rosenberg R, Beard CB. Vector-borne infections. *Emerg Infect Dis*. 2011;17:769–770.

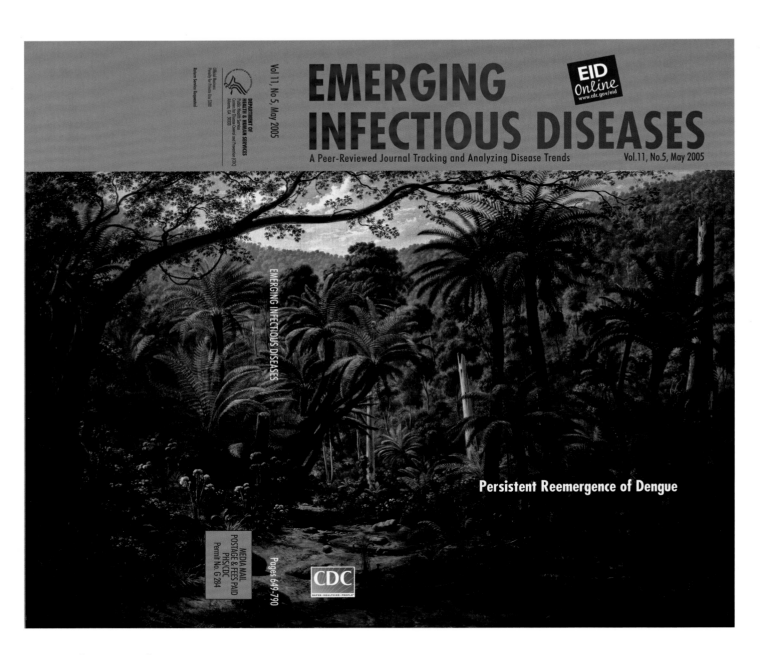

EMERGING
INFECTIOUS DISEASES
A Peer-Reviewed Journal Tracking and Analyzing Disease Trends
Vol.11, No.5, May 2005

EID Online
www.cdc.gov/eid

Vol 11, No 5, May 2005

DEPARTMENT OF
HEALTH & HUMAN SERVICES
Public Health Service
Centers for Disease Control and Prevention (CDC)
Atlanta, GA 30333

Official Business
Penalty for Private Use $300

Return Service Requested

EMERGING INFECTIOUS DISEASES

MEDIA MAIL
POSTAGE & FEES PAID
PHS/CDC
Permit No. G-284

Pages 649-790

Persistent Reemergence of Dengue

CDC
SAFER·HEALTHIER·PEOPLE™

Emerg. Infect. Dis., Vol. 11, No. 5, May 2005

LANDSCAPE TRANSFORMATION AND DISEASE EMERGENCE

During his long ocean passage to Australia in 1852, Eugene von Guérard reported that conditions were far from ideal, and "meals were late and bad." He had boarded a sailing ship at Gravesend, England, to seek his fortune in Victoria. At the gold fields of Ballarat, he described mining as "arduous at first" and causing "much backache and blistering of hands." His gold mining efforts in Ballarat and environs were unsuccessful, and after a year, he abandoned the venture. Even so, he had struck gold. His illustrated diaries chronicled the history of the region, the harsh life of the gold digger, and the scarring of landscape from gold mining. He opened a studio in Melbourne, soon to become the most important Australian artist of his day.

The son of an artist and court painter, von Guérard was born in Vienna, Austria. He toured Italy with his father and lived in Rome for a while, where he became familiar with the work of famed French landscapists Claude Lorraine and Nicholas Poussin. Later, he studied landscape painting at the Dusseldorf Academy, where he was influenced by German romanticism—a movement that also dwelled on the visual aspects of nature. During his 30 years in Australia, he became a renowned landscape painter, as well as teacher and honorary curator at the National Gallery in Victoria. He died in London, where he had settled near the end of his life.

The 1850s gold rush that lured von Guérard to Victoria coincided with a revived interest in landscape painting, particularly in Australia and the United States (the Hudson River school). In the midst of 19th-century urbanization grew a longing to connect with nature. Travelers sought areas of untouched wilderness, and artists labored to bring exotic freshness to the homebound. From his studio in Melbourne, von Guérard traveled to and explored many regions, among them timbered Illawarra and Tasmania, seeking the picturesque and generating drawings for his monumental landscape paintings.

At Illawarra, von Guérard was able to capture, in minute detail, the character of local flora: cabbage palms, ferns, fig trees, and multiple varieties of vines within the dark green tones of the dense Australian forest. Meticulous geographic, geologic, and ecosystem markers lend his artistic work historical importance as backdrop to subsequent transformation of the landscape by widespread mining and population growth.

In a letter to the Melbourne newspaper *The Argus* in 1870, von Guérard explained that he painted "with the greatest desire to imitate nature" and sought to capture not only her details but also her "poetical feelings." Descriptive and emotional, his elaborate artistic observations imbued the physical world with inner life quite apart from human society. Like many of his contemporaries (e.g., American painter Frederic Church), von Guérard was influenced by prominent German naturalist Alexander von Humboldt (1769–1859), who advocated a "mutual reinforcement of art and science." In this context, topographic detail was acceptable in paintings only if motivated and sustained by emotional connection and personal relevance. Landscape painting was a way to express love of nature. And nature was constantly changing, driven by forces that shaped it throughout the eons.

Ferntree Gully in the Dandenong Ranges was hailed a masterpiece in its day. A lush mountain panorama, this painting excels in its faithful depiction of both the forest and the trees. Balanced and lyrical, the work is a romantic rendering of pure, unadulterated nature. The scene is carefully structured: background fully outlined, center well lit, and foreground intentionally shaded to frame the cloistered center. Each leaf is described in detail.

A broad path leads inward for a better look at the botanical life nearby as well as the treed horizon afar. A couple of lyrebirds walk the brush, their ancient silhouettes outlined against the grounds sheltering their fare of insects, myriapods, and snails. Curving fern tops and tree branches create a circular feeling as the eye moves from dark to light, from mountaintop to forest floor, from live greenery to fallen tree limbs and skeletal trunks, recounting a natural cycle of death and regeneration.

Von Guérard provided a respectful glimpse at unspoiled wilderness. His artistic eye scanned the exotic flora and through the bucolic stillness saw the real Arcadia, a goldmine of natural elements in constant change.

The semitropical rainforest idyll witnessed by von Guérard in Illawarra repeats itself in tropical and subtropical regions around the globe. Under a canopy of green, away from direct light, rain, and wind, moisture seeps down or hangs in midair, creating a fertile environment for propagation and growth. Along with fern spores, wildlife and microbial life are beneficiaries of the gullies' hothouse. Tiny creatures of the forest and blood-sucking insects, nature's fine detail, populate the underbrush—among them, mosquitoes, which feed on wild animals and thrive in this habitat.

As human development encroaches on the forest and urbanization transforms the native environment, mosquitoes become able to travel to all global destinations. These adaptable insects, some of them vectors of dengue viruses, have become anthropophilic, domesticated, and dangerous to humans. Environmental change affects nature's cycle, once more frustrating efforts to disrupt the persistent reemergence of dengue and other tropical diseases.

Bibliography

Calisher C. Persistent reemergence of dengue. *Emerg Infect Dis.* 2005;11:738–739.

Clark J, Whitelaw B. *Golden Summers: Heidelberg and Beyond.* Sydney, Australia: International Cultural Corporation of Australia; 1986.

The garden of New South Wales; http://www.michaelorgan.org.au; accessed March 30, 2005.

Thomas D. Australian art. In: *The Encyclopedia of Visual Art.* Danbury, CT: Grolier Educational Corporation; 1983.

EMERGING
EID Online
www.cdc.gov/eid

INFECTIOUS DISEASES

A Peer-Reviewed Journal Tracking and Analyzing Disease Trends

Vol.11, No.11, November 2005

Avian Influenza

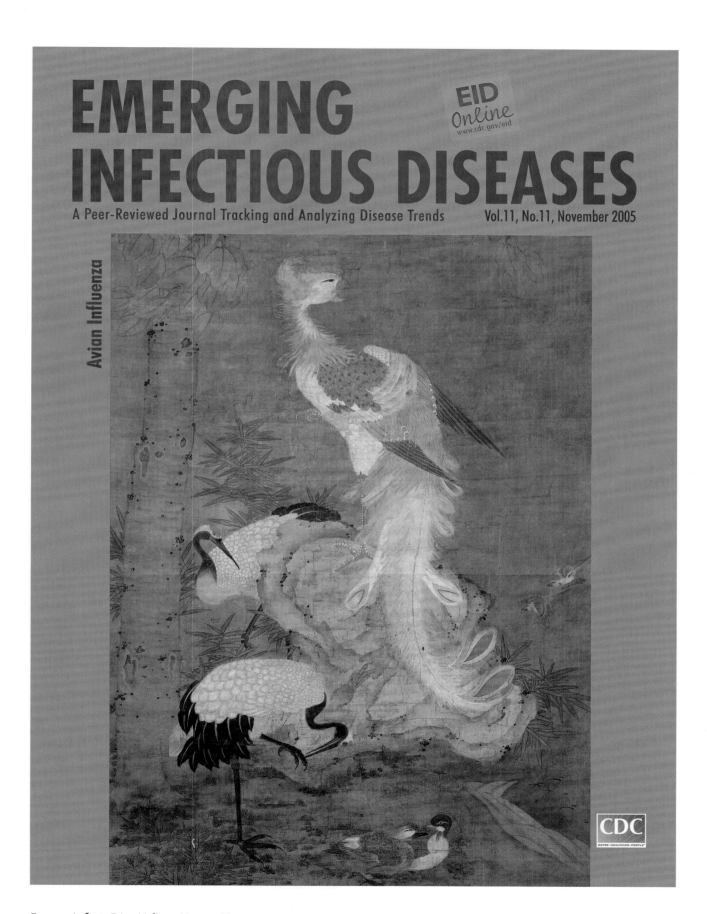

CDC
SAFER·HEALTHIER·PEOPLE

PHOENIX AND FOWL—BIRDS OF A FEATHER

A treasured aviary, the vast collection of bird paintings in Chinese art, reflects long-standing global fascination with our feathered friends. Balanced on two legs, like humans, and able to fly and swim, birds have been viewed as an engineering miracle in the East and West and have been studied by artists and scientists alike.

Traditional Chinese painting goes back 6,000 years to the Neolithic period and is found on early pottery decorated with brush images of humans and animals. Painting of flowers and birds originated on this primitive pottery, as well as on bronze and silk adorned with simple but brightly colored designs. The genre, which is seen throughout Chinese art history, flourished during the Song dynasty (1101–1125).

During the Yuan dynasty (1279–1368), the Mongol wars and general turmoil under Genghis Khan overshadowed a strong artistic legacy enriched by diverse foreign influences. The period saw suspension of artists' and intellectuals' rights and retreat to traditional styles of painting. Need for greater artistic expression coincided with the return of native rule during the Ming dynasty.

The Ming dynasty (1368–1644) was a time of cultural restoration and expansion for the Chinese, a "scholar's culture" of thriving literary and artistic communities populated by writers, poets, and artists, many of them outstanding masters with extraordinary skills and breadth. Revived interest in local culture was often expressed in landscape images of mountains or other nature scenes painted on scrolls. Monochrome and color woodblock printing developed and advanced at this time, as did porcelain production and diversification. Yet artists worked primarily in a revival of Song academic styles, prescribed by a conservative court for its glorification and prestige.

Genius is the most important quality in a painter, knowledge comes next, and "the single brush stroke is the source of all things," wrote painter and member of the Ming royal house, Shitao (1642–1707). Unlike canvas, silk, which was used in painting even before paper was invented, was unforgiving of errors and required exceptional skill and confidence. Many renowned Chinese painters were also expert calligraphers and poets, who often made literary references in landscape painting, emphasizing the connection between disciplines and adding complexity to the work.

Phoenix and Birds exhibits many of the qualities of Ming dynasty silk scroll painting. The narrative content: Five Human Relationships Represented by Five Different Birds is expressed with surely executed lines and subtle colors in vertical format. Shadow, light, and proportion are used to create a third dimension. A central figure, the phoenix, dominates the scene. This legendary bird, part of global mythology, is described here in the Chinese tradition. Like the dragon, with which it is often associated, the phoenix, or fenghuang, exemplifies the union of yin and yang (polar opposites complementing each other in nature and underlying order within the universe).

In some legends, the fenghuang is created from desirable parts of other creatures: cock's beak, swallow's face, fowl's forehead, snake's neck, goose's breast, tortoise's back, stag's hind, fish's tail. Its song reflects the notes of the musical scale, its feathers five fundamental colors, its figure the celestial bodies: head symbolizes the sky; eyes, the sun; back, the moon; feet, the earth; tail, the planets. This emperor of birds is anchored on a rock, its royal plumes and fearless stare signaling preeminence. Below are two cranes, symbols of wisdom and longevity. They seem aware of their surroundings and of two other waterfowl fraternizing in the foreground.

In this harmonious bird scene, the unknown artist injects a measure of Confucian values, the need for each creature to act not singly but in connection with others, through five relationships: parent–child, husband–wife, sibling–sibling, friend–friend, ruler–subject, in networks of individual persons, the family, the state, the universe. This conglomeration of myth and Confucian wisdom within the Asian tradition has timeless implications. And in today's context, troubled by the specter of pandemic avian flu, *Phoenix and Birds* seems prophetic.

The bird ensemble captures issues at the heart of our current predicament: unknown pathogen origins, exotic composites of unlikely elements, increasing complexity, vast public health implications. The imperial phoenix with its patchwork beauty, perched high on the mount is not much different from the frolicking cranes or the humble fowl crouching anonymously in the foreground. All participate in nature's play.

More than the sum of its unlikely parts, the phoenix recalls the flu virus and its wild recombination. Less conspicuously, the migrating waterfowl signal this species' importance as reservoir hosts and dissemination agents, bringing the virus to creatures absent from this painting (domestic poultry, swine). The circle is complete as new opportunities arise for recombination with local mammalian strains to form a new virus with pandemic potential. Confucian relationships meet nature's whim.

Bibliography

Consulate General of The People's Republic of China in Los Angeles. Chinese painting. Available at: http://losangeles.china-consulate.org/eng/culture/acc/t83968.htm. Accessed April 24, 2013.

Hobson RL, Binyon L, Sirén O, et al. *The Romance of Chinese Art*. New York, NY: Garden City Publishing; 1936.

Metropolitan Museum of Art. Ming dynasty (1368–1644). Available at: http://www.metmuseum.org/toah/hd/ming/hd_ming.htm. Accessed April 25, 2013.

ThinkQuest. Confucianism. Available at: http://library.thinkquest.org/12255/temple/confucianism.html. Accessed April 24, 2013.

EMERGING
INFECTIOUS DISEASES

A Peer-Reviewed Journal Tracking and Analyzing Disease Trends

Vol.11, No.7, July 2005

EID Online
www.cdc.gov/eid

Global Wildlife Trade

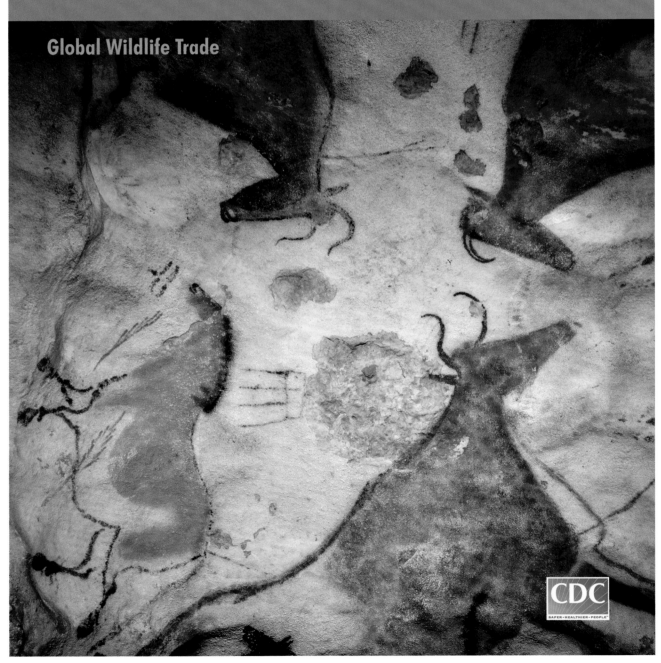

CDC
SAFER · HEALTHIER · PEOPLE™

PALEOLITHIC MURALS AND THE GLOBAL WILDLIFE TRADE

"Antiquities are history defaced," argued Renaissance philosopher Francis Bacon in *The Advancement of Learning*; they are "remnants of history which . . . escaped the shipwreck of time." These remnants, battered by the elements and scattered around the globe, are all we have to piece together human heritage. In recent years, radiocarbon dating techniques (e.g., accelerator mass spectrometry) have allowed us to date samples of pigment from cave paintings and not rely solely on evidence from surrounding artifacts. These techniques shed light on the chronology and evolution of prehistoric art and show that cave painting began much earlier than believed, as early as the Upper Paleolithic period.

The Paleolithic period (Old Stone Age), the earliest stretch of human history 2 million years ago, saw the development of the human species. Nomadic hunters and gatherers, who lived in caves and crafted tools out of stone, progressed during the last ice age to communal hunting, constructed shelters, and belief systems. The Upper Paleolithic (end of Old Stone Age) marks humanity's cognitive and cultural, as well as artistic, beginnings.

When, why, and how precisely humans moved from rote tool making to symbolic self-expression is not known. Evidence gathered in the past 200 years indicates that graphic activity (figurative and nonfigurative marks) began as early as 40,000 years ago, preceding the development of agriculture. It coincided with human migration around the globe, the production of implements from multiple materials, and the building of simple machines. Images carved, etched, or painted on stone, clay, bone, horn, ivory, or antler were found in Africa, Australia, the Middle East, and Europe, and portable sculptures of animal and human figures were more common and widespread than cave paintings.

The first discoveries of Paleolithic painting, which were greeted with skepticism and disbelief, were made around 1835 in France and Switzerland and later in Spain, Australia, South Africa, and other places. The western edges of the Massif Central region of France and the northern slopes of the Pyrenees are dotted with more than a hundred Paleolithic caves, among them renowned Lascaux. Naturally blocked for thousands of years, these deep caves maintained sufficiently stable temperature and humidity to preserve, untouched, not only paintings but also footprints and handprints of their inhabitants. After the discovery of Lascaux in 1940, environmental conditions changed. A fungus (*Fusarium*) began to grow inside the cave, and algae spread on the floor, walls, and ceiling, threatening the integrity of the paintings. The threat was contained, but access to the public was curtailed.

The cavern "gave onto a steep slope, slippery and slimy . . . with flakes of worked flint of poor quality, some fragments of reindeer horns and many pieces of conifer charcoal," recalled speleologist Abbé Breuil about the initial opening to Lascaux. The ground was different 17,000 years ago. The cave had sunk and was difficult to reach, the entrance obscured by millennia of erosion and sediment.

The dark sanctuary contained a network of passages, caverns, and shafts, later named Great Hall of the Bulls, Painted Gallery, Chamber of Engravings, Chamber of Felines, and Shaft of the Dead Man. Uneven wall and ceiling surfaces sported enigmatic scratches, smudges, and combinations of dots and grids, as well as drawings and painted figures whose narrative meaning had been rendered unfathomable by the passage of time.

Mineral pigments (ochre, charcoal, iron oxide, hematite, manganese) were ground into animal fat and applied with brushes or were blown through hollow sticks. The artists, working in confined, possibly dangerous space, under unsteady or flickering light from a torch or oil lamp, incorporated distortions and shadows in the design, along with soot.

As if suddenly awakened from extended hibernation, herds of aurochs, horses, chamois, ibexes, bison, stags, and rhinoceroses rush en masse on the cave walls. Large wild beasts, drawn not from life but from the imagination, populate free-flowing compositions in coordinated movement with each other. Their bodies, intently outlined and punctuated with color, at once realistic and stylized, conform to the contours of the cave, the cracks and imperfections of which are often incorporated in the drawing. Anatomical details betray familiarity with the animals, as well as observational and artistic skill. Proportions are mostly accurate, except for the heads, which tend to be small, and the horns, which are sometimes exaggerated. Unrestricted and unbound, the beasts frolic on the dark walls, at times overlapping as they gallop toward or away from each other.

A strong "occluding contour," an essential silhouette, is etched or painted on the hard surfaces. The silhouette, often the only graphic, boasts a prominent cervico-dorsal line, in profile. And this line is at times the only line, as if part of the animal is drawn to suggest the whole. Even though figures are presented in profile, distinctive details (horns or hooves) have an independent, "twisted" orientation.

Large animals are the protagonists. Humans, if present at all, are stick figures, masked or headless, crudely drawn, stiff and nonexpressive, their puzzling presence possibly symbolic and secondary. We do not know whether these murals represent early social interactions (the hunt, sacred rites, tribal ceremonies); hallucinogenic imagination inflamed by fumes in unventilated caves; unknown primitive rituals; or simply artistic compulsion. Yet this preferential and exuberant treatment of animals suggests on the part of our ancestors inexplicable fascination with wildlife.

As far back as the Paleolithic age, humans have lived in close proximity with animals, associating not only with those they could domesticate but also with wild and dangerous beasts. Encounters contained an element of risk, for humans were injured or killed as much as nourished or entertained. The enigmatic portrayal of large, wild beasts on the walls and ceiling at Lascaux suggests a complex early relationship that went beyond the necessities of food or fiber. In our time, interaction with animals continues to encompass cohabitation at all levels, including the microbial. Encounters, compounded by increased travel and trade, still involve risks as well as benefits. And even though we are less likely to be injured or killed by animals, the exotic pathogens living and traveling with them counterbalance amusement and companionship with illness and death.

Bibliography

Bednarik RG. The first stirrings of creation. *UNESCO Cour.* 1998;51:4.

Brodrick HB. *Father of Prehistory, Abbe Henri Breuil: His Life and Times.* New York, NY: H. Wolff; 1963.

Karesh WB, Cook RA, Bennett EL, Newcomb J. Wildlife trade and global disease emergence. *Emerg Infect Dis.* 2005;11:1000–1003.

Valladas H. Direct radiocarbon dating of prehistoric cave paintings by accelerator mass spectrometry. *Meas Sci Technol.* 2003;14:1487–1492.

Vol 11, No 3, March 2005

EID Online
www.cdc.gov/eid

EMERGING
INFECTIOUS DISEASES

A Peer-Reviewed Journal Tracking and Analyzing Disease Trends   Vol.11, No.3, March 2005

Ebola Virus Antibodies in Dogs

CDC

Pages 361-518

MEDIA MAIL
POSTAGE & FEES PAID
PHS/CDC
Permit No. G-284

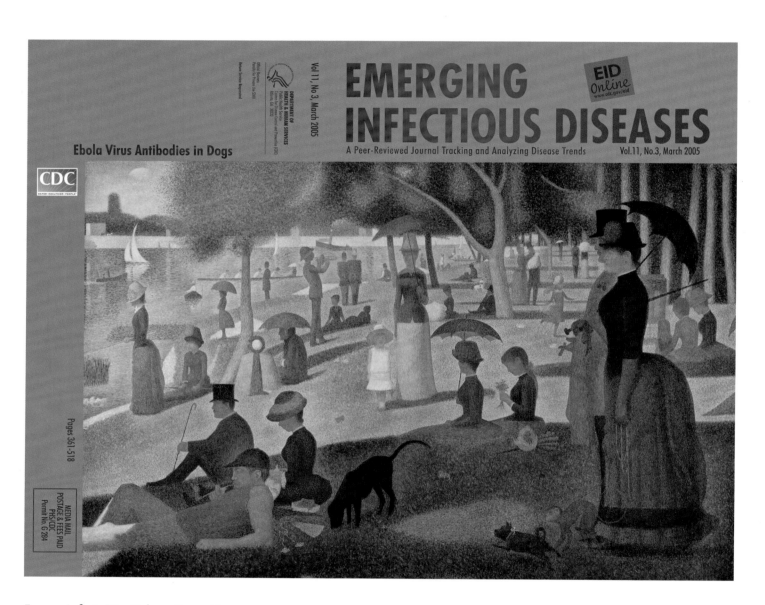

Emerg. Infect. Dis., Vol. 11, No. 3, Mar. 2005

OPTICS AND BIOLOGIC CONNECTEDNESS

"It is this passion for beautiful colors that makes us paint as we do . . . and not the love of the 'dot,' as foolish people say," wrote painter Paul Signac in his journal. He was defending the art movement started by his good friend and fellow artist George Seurat and built upon by Signac, himself, Camille Pissarro, and others. This movement, divisionism or pointillism, was Seurat's artistic contribution during a brief but extraordinary life.

Parisian from a middle-class family, tall, and handsome, Seurat enjoyed a comfortable life and proper education. He showed early talent for drawing, studied sculpture, and attended the prestigious École des Beaux-Arts. A competent photographer, he became interested in the workings of light, particularly in black-and-white images. This interest grew as he studied optics and the processes at work on the silver particles of photographic film. During his art studies, particularly under the tutelage of a student of Ingres, he came to believe in a systematic approach to art.

Nicknamed *le notaire* (the notary) for his immaculate attention to his appearance, Seurat was temperamentally suited for a scientific approach to art. Idiosyncratically bent toward order and control and gifted with formidable observational skills, patience, concentration, and painstaking adherence to detail, he embarked on a style of painting based on color and structure that was cerebral and calculated.

Like the impressionists, Seurat was interested in the relationship between natural light and the application of paint, only he wanted to create an impression not on the canvas but in the mind of the viewer. Influenced by the work of French chemist Michel-Eugène Chevreul (1786–1889), he believed that next to each other, colors appear as dissimilar as possible, both in optical composition and tonal value. Seurat's color theory, in which the viewer plays a key role in perception, influenced the development of modern art.

His artistic goal, Seurat once said, was to show "modern people, in their essential traits, move about as if on friezes, and place them on canvases organized by harmonies of color, by directions of the tones in harmony with the lines, and by the directions of the lines." In his best known work, images are tightly structured as if on a grid, the figures systematically placed in relation to each other in permanent, nonnegotiable arrangements. Pure color is used directly from the tube, in static "points" clearly separate but intended to merge in the viewer's eye, producing a confluent image brighter than any achieved with brushstrokes. Like many scientific experiments, Seurat's daring process had unexpected results. The points remained visible, akin to tesserae in a mosaic, but produced a shimmering translucent effect.

A Sunday Afternoon on the Island of La Grande Jatte is Seurat's masterpiece and one of the best-known works of the 19th century. The placid scene in an island park on the Seine shows a local crowd during a moment of leisure outdoors. Seurat's version of this commonplace event is revolutionary. As figures register in the viewer's eye, they seem suspended in mid-moment, levitating yet permanently fixed. Prototypes rather than likenesses, they represent workers in shirt sleeves, fashionable couples, children at play, soldiers in uniform. Seurat did not dwell on their faces, nor did he offer anything but their frontal or profile forms—classical, refined, distinct, balanced, and frozen in time. The iconic setup, like backdrop in a period drama, impassionedly places people, animals, and objects in a suddenly interrupted scene, creating a spellbinding visual effect.

As much interested in the science as in the art of painting, Seurat used figures as scene building blocks. Elegantly curved and grouped in harmonious ensembles, the figures are isolated from each other and detached from the beauty around them. And like separate dots of color, they do not fully blend, their shimmering presence only a means to a perfect artistic end.

Seurat's own life embodied the personal isolation seen in *La Grande Jatte*. Even though surrounded by friends and supported by family, he was intensely private, even secretive, about his affairs. His parents did not know that he had a child until he was taken ill, possibly with diphtheria. He died precipitously at age 31, while hard at his innovative work. Signac encapsulated his friend's achievement: "He surveyed the scene and has made these very important contributions: his black and white, his harmony of lines, his composition, his contrast and harmony of color, even his frames. What more can you ask of a painter?"

Seurat was not interested in the emotional or evolutionary connectedness of the crowd in *La Grande Jatte*. The nannies, belles and beaux, the playful pet monkey, even the stray dog foraging picnic crumbs in the foreground, are locked into themselves. Had Seurat been interested in biologic rather than optical accuracy, he might have ventured beyond visual perception of the crowd on the lawn. And between the dots, he might have found invisible connectedness, the glue that binds humans, monkeys, stray dogs, and vegetation. Impervious to optics and inaccessible to the naked eye, biologic connectedness abounds.

Around the world, as in *La Grande Jatte*, scrounging animals share the landscape with humans. Along with scraps of food, they gather data that properly transcribed can be valuable. In African forest villages, loose dogs living near hunters and eating dead animals become exposed to Ebola and carry antibodies to the virus. Their destinies intertwined with ours in a way inaccessible to Seurat, the dogs may become predictors of human disease as their serologic status signals the presence of virus in the community.

Bibliography
Allela L. Ebola virus antibody prevalence in dogs and human risk. *Emerg Infect Dis.* 2005;11:385–390.
Broude N, ed. *Seurat in Perspective.* Englewood Cliffs, NJ: Prentice-Hall; 1978.
Hunter S. Georges Seurat. In *Modern Art.* New York, NY: Harry N. Abrams; 1992:27.
Vora SK. Death of Seurat. *Emerg Infect Dis.* 2005;11:162–166.

Human Demographics and Behavior

"Others will have greater skill for getting the breath of life to spring from bronze more fluidly. . . . But as for you, Roman, remember to impose your power upon nations. Your art is to decree the rules of peace, to spare the vanquished and subdue the vainglorious," advised Virgil in the *Aeneid*, placing himself in the service of imperial ideology. This was the reign of Augustus, the first and among the most influential of Roman emperors, who more than 2,000 years ago enlisted literature and the arts in support of the new order.

In the Augustan era, sculpture still showed the idealism of Hellenic models, even relief sculpture: shallow three-dimensional carvings on arches, friezes, altars, and other flat areas of temples and public buildings. But the content of reliefs favored the historical and commemorative, intending to narrate in detail triumphant military campaigns and promote the goals of the Empire. In his *Ars Poetica*, Horace supported this philosophy, as he argued for the superiority of painting over any other form of communication to affect and manipulate: "Less vividly is the mind stirred by what finds entrance through the ears than by what is brought before the trusty eyes, and what the spectator can see for himself." Public art of the Empire aimed to "write conquerors and conquered in one community."

Contiguous panels of the relief used on a cover of *Emerging Infectious Diseases* have the feel of narrative stream. During the census proceedings, a collection of citizens, among them military men serving as guards, are taking part in a religious rite. The sacrifice, whose purpose was purification, was performed at state ceremonies, during agricultural festivals to drive out evil from the fields and purify new crops, as atonement for ritual errors, before military campaigns, and at the conclusion of the census.

The census was the first and principal duty of the Roman censors, high magistrates in charge of this 5-yearly activity. To carry out the census and the purifications that concluded it, they had the power of summoning the people to the Campus Martius, each tribe separately, by public crier. Each paterfamilias appeared in person to account for himself, his family, and his property upon oath, "declared from the heart." A person voluntarily absent from the census was considered *incensus* and risked imprisonment and death.

"It is so hard to find out the truth of anything by looking at the record of the past," wrote Plutarch; "The process of time obscures the truth of former times, and even contemporaneous writers disguise and twist the truth out of malice or flattery." Even art can be used for promotion and persuasion. Yet this census-taking relief, a glimpse of Roman life, did more than serve the purposes of the state. It witnessed one of the foundation stones of Roman civilization; a ritual special to the Romans for it symbolized their status as a *populus*, a people, capable of collective action.

Human behavior, individual or collective, difficult as it may be to categorize, is key to disease emergence. Frida Kahlo's *Self-Portrait with Monkey* frames the painter's close relationship with her pet. The portrait also alludes to another relationship, one that the painter and her contemporaries were not aware of, the philogenetic kinship with her pet and the caution prescribed by this kinship. More recently, increased popularity of exotic animals (monkeys, rodents, hedgehogs) as pets compromises the integrity of natural cycles. Exotic pets relocated from their indigenous environments to other areas carry with them frequently uncharacterized or unknown zoonotic pathogens. Prairie dogs, the most social members of the squirrel family, have made their settlements from Montana to Texas and in higher elevations of the Mojave, Great Basin, and Chihuahuan deserts, posing little risk to humans as long as nature and its endemic zoonoses were in balance. Georgia O'Keeffe's *Scull with Calico Roses* reminds how relocation of animals has proven perilous to both animal and human communities and has raised the specter of interspecies transmission of infectious agents, among them those that cause dangerous infections like tularemia and monkeypox.

Human susceptibility to infection can influence changes in a pathogen and its transmission pathways. Human infections resulting from impaired immune defenses are "opportunistic" since they are caused by microbes that "take advantage" of a person's weakened immune status. Changes influencing human susceptibility to infection include increases in the use of immunosuppressive drugs and in the number of patients with compromised immune systems, particularly those receiving cancer chemotherapy or undergoing organ transplantation. Because aging and malnutrition can have the same compromising effect on the immune system, the elderly and indigent are more susceptible to many infections, including foodborne and diarrheal diseases, which in turn increase the severity of malnutrition. Giovanni Battista Tiepolo's *Bust of an Old Man* sheds light on this neglected group, the elderly, who are not often the subject of art.

Antimicrobial-drug resistance is linked to human demographics and behavior. Treating resistant infections often requires expensive and toxic alternative drugs, prolongs hospital stays, and increases risk for death. Development of new drugs is hampered by lack of new agents and by market forces. Demand for new drugs is greatest in areas of the world that can least afford to support new drug development. High levels of pesticides in agriculture contribute to resistance in insects, some of which carry human disease. Pesticide resistance, as well as the legal restrictions placed on pesticide use, hinders efforts to control disease carriers. Our well-tested, heretofore reliable drugs against malaria are losing their effectiveness. *Krishna Storms the Citadel of Naraka* is a metaphorical description of the monumental forces involved in antimicrobial-drug resistance.

New diseases emerge in different parts of the world at any time and without warning. Predicting where and when is very difficult. But gathering clues, particularly those related to human demographics and behavior and to human–animal interaction, can help resolve the public health puzzles and draw attention to problem areas. Meanwhile, with some infections, such as SARS, treatment has to be administered before all the pieces of the puzzle have been assembled. The old measures of quarantine and infection control are challenged by new environmental, social, and scientific developments. Francisco José de Goya y Lucientes's *Self-portrait with Doctor Arrieta* illuminates this point.

"We are all, so far as we inherit the civilizations of Europe, still citizens of the Roman Empire," wrote T. S. Eliot, poet and critic of modern European culture. And while his words may not have universal application, they do call attention to Roman legacy in some of our practices. Certainly we relate to the census. In ancient Rome, the practice served to count citizens and assess military strength and tax revenue. In public health, it helps calculate population density. The number of humans, animals, plants, wildlife, and vectors per unit area influences the spread of communicable diseases and their impact, a tax of its own. And "census numbers" of domestic and wild animals, the denominators used to calculate attack, birth, and death rates, can be strong predictors of zoonotic disease. Once again in the words of T. S. Eliot, "withered stumps of time . . . told upon the walls" uncover uncommon denominators.

Bibliography

Capes WW. *The Early Empire.* London, England: Longman, Green, and Co.; 1897.

Horace. Ars poetica. In: Hardison OB Jr, Goldern L, trans-eds. *Horace for Students of Literature: The "Ars Poetica" and Its Tradition.* Gainesville, FL: University Press of Florida; 1995.

O'Keeffe G. About myself. In: *Georgia O'Keeffe: Exhibition of Pils and Pastels.* New York: An American Place; 1939.

Potter P. Uncommon denominators. *Emerg Infect Dis.* 2007; 13:1974–1975.

Roman society. Roman life. Available at: http://www.roman-empire.net/society/society.html. Accessed October 3, 2007.

Virgil. *The Aeneid.* Fitzgerald R, trans. New York, NY: Vintage Books; 1990.

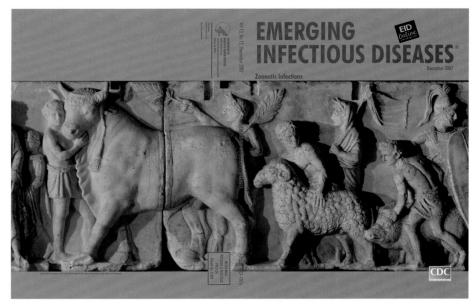

Zoonotic Infections; http://dx.doi.org/10.3201/eid1312.AC1312

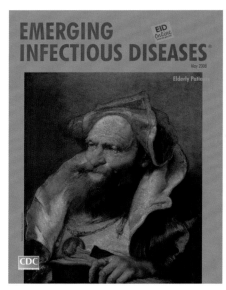

Elderly Patients; http://dx.doi.
org/10.3201/eid1405.AC1405

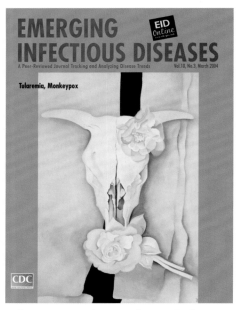

Tularemia, Monkeypox; http://dx.doi.
org/10.3201/eid1003.AC1003

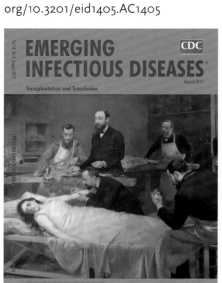

Transplantation and Transfusion; http://
dx.doi.org/10.3201/eid1808.AC1808

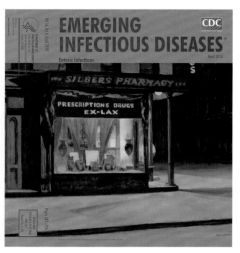

Enteric Infections; http://dx.doi.
org/10.3201/eid1604.AC1604

EMERGING
INFECTIOUS DISEASES®

Vector-borne Infections

March 2010

A FLEA HAS SMALLER FLEAS THAT ON HIM PREY; AND THESE HAVE SMALLER STILL TO BITE 'EM, AND SO PROCEED AD INFINITUM[1]

"There was no doubt that this poor man was mad, but there is something in the madness of this man which interests me more than the sanity of Lord Byron and Walter Scott," remarked William Wordsworth about his fellow poet William Blake. Blake's own claims to outlandish visions added fuel to rumors of his insanity. As a mere child, he saw God "put his head through the window" and on another occasion, "a tree filled with angels, bright angelic wings bespangling every bough like stars." Later in life, when faced with the death of a younger sibling, he saw this brother's spirit "clapping its hands for joy."

Blake was a Londoner, born in a spacious old home at 28 Broad Street, Golden Square, the son of a hosier. He never went to school and throughout his life was glad to have escaped formal education: "Improvement makes strait roads; but the crooked roads without Improvement are roads of genius." His family indulged his talents. "As soon as the child's hand could hold a pencil it began to scrawl rough likenesses of man or beast and make timid copies of all the prints he came near." At age 10 he was sent to a fashionable preparatory school for young artists, and at 14, he was apprenticed to Basire, engraver to the Society of Antiquaries, who sent him to draw old monuments, especially at Westminster Abbey. His love of Gothic art dates from this time.

He delighted in the linear nature of monuments for he believed "firm and determinate lineaments unbroken by shadows" to be the essence of art. He abhorred chiaroscuro, the art of Venice and Flanders, because its interplay of light and shadow blurred outlines. Linear style was also characteristic of religious art. The spirits he drew, Blake insisted, should be "organized" within determinate and bounding form. Admiration of Greek antiquities and mythology also nurtured his style and subject matter.

For a man who never strayed far from his home town, he became very cultured in the visual arts. In his prime a distinguished printer, painter, poet, and musician, as well as prophet and iconoclast, Blake took education in his own hands. He learned Greek, Latin, and Hebrew to appreciate the classics in the original and invented his own engraving and color preservation techniques. He combined his facility with the word and brush in "illuminated printing," a technique rooted in the Middle Ages, to bring poetry to the reader through the eye of the poet's own imagination. Eccentric and nonconformist, he associated with radical thinkers, among them Thomas Paine and Mary Wollstonecraft.

Blake's work was on a small scale and often contained in the pages of books. But his imaginings were boundless. "He who does not imagine in stronger and better lineaments and in stronger and better light than his perishing and mortal eye can see does not imagine at all." To him the great art of the world depicted not that seen by the "mortal eye" but a more perfect imagined form. His idiosyncratic

---

1 Jonathan Swift, "On Poetry: A Rhapsody" (1733).

approach to life and the individuality of his craft defy labels. While his work places him solidly among the Romantics, some have labeled him a forerunner of modern anarchism.

Many spirits or ghosts Blake drew seemed to derive from his Gothic studies; others were of kings or queens. In *The Ghost of a Flea*, the ghost seems that of a demon. This miniature was part of a series of "visionary heads," commissioned by his friend John Varley, landscape painter and astrologer, who believed in spirits but was unable to see them. He was drawn to Blake, who professed to live with them. The two would meet and try to summon spirits of historical or mythologic figures, and if they appeared, Blake would draw them. They were angels, Voltaire, Moses, and the flea, which told them that "Fleas were inhabited by the souls of such men as were by nature blood thirsty to excess."

"I called on him one evening and found Blake more than usually excited," Varley reported. "He had seen a wonderful thing—the ghost of a flea!" "And did you make a drawing of him?" Varley asked. "I wish I had," Blake responded, "but I shall, if he appears again! . . . There he comes! His eager tongue whisking out of this mouth." Varley gave him paper and a pencil to draw the portrait. "I felt convinced by his mode of proceedings that he had a real image before him, for he left off, and began on another part of the paper, to make a separate drawing of the mouth of the flea, which the spirit having opened, he was prevented from proceeding with the first sketch, till he had closed it."

Varley described the conception as a "naked figure with a strong body and a short neck—with burning eyes which long for moisture, and a face worthy of a murderer holding a bloody cup in its clawed hands, out of which it seems eager to drink. . . . I never saw any shape so strange, nor did I ever see any colouring so curiously splendid—a kind of glistening green and dusky gold, beautifully varnished."

Both in his poetry and his art, Blake often personified death, war, famine, and other abstractions, ascribing them faces and human characteristics. The ghost of his flea is muscular, part human part reptile, loaded with symbolic clues of its nature and character. The creature strides theatrically across a stage framed by opulent drapes and sprinkled with stars—Blake's friend and supporter John Linnell made a copy of this drawing for *Zodiacal Physiognomy*, as a sign of Gemini.

The left hand holds an acorn, the right a thorn. The massive frame scarred by a protruding spine supports a small head, vaguely alluding to the shape of a flea. On the floor near the feet, an insect, the physical embodiment, completes the portrait. Despite claims to a visionary source, this flea recalls the imps of Henry Fuseli (1741–1825), another painter of monsters, and some of Blake's previous work. It could also have been informed by the drawings of early microscopist Robert Hooke (1635–1703), whose illustration of a flea in his book *Micrographia* described it as "adorn'd with a curiously polish'd suite of sable Armour, neatly jointed."

"It's God. / I'd know him from Blake's picture anywhere," Robert Frost's Eve said in "Masque of Reason." Whether he was drawing the Almighty or a tiny insect, Blake captured and uncloaked the unadulterated character of the subject. And whatever the source of his inspiration, it lit and portrayed this character in all its purity.

Not fooled by the tiny creature he tossed on the scene as a reference, Blake knew and spelled out its horrific nature. And he was not alone. The flea was notorious for its pestiferous qualities. They did not escape the attention of Jonathan Swift: "The vermin only tease and pinch / Their foes superior by an inch." John Donne (1572–1631) had exploited the flea's blood-drinking habits in his immortal plea to a mistress, acknowledging the importance of fluid exchange, before the possibility of contagion even entered the equation, "Me it suck'd first, and now sucks thee, / And in this flea our two bloods mingled bee."

The perpetual struggle against these pests inspires poetry to this day: "Fleas / Adam / had 'em." The incongruous imbalance between their size and their impact on humanity, shown in no less than their deadly connection with the history of Black Death, is now fully understood. Fleas are known for the vectors of disease they are, spreading in addition to bubonic plague, murine or fleaborne typhus and other rickettsioses in new areas, and still tormenting and killing humans, despite improved diagnostic techniques and treatments. Swift would see no humor in the ad infinitum emergence of novel spotted fever strains causing disease in yet more areas. He could not have known that microorganisms, such as rickettsia, infect fleas and through them spread to other animals, in fact becoming what he had lightly referred to as the fleas of fleas.

Bibliography

Adjemian J, Parks S, McElroy K. Murine typhus in Austin, Texas, USA, 2008. *Emerg Infect Dis.* 2010;16:412–417.

Bentley GE, Bentley G Jr. *William Blake: The Critical Heritage.* London, England: Routledge; 1995.

Gilchrist A. *The Life of William Blake.* London, England: McMillan; 1863.

Kelly PJ, Lucas H, Eremeeva ME, et al. *Rickettsia felis,* West Indies. *Emerg Infect Dis.* 2010;16:570–571.

Myrone M. *The Blake Book.* London, England: Tate Gallery; 2007.

Raine K. *William Blake.* New York, NY: Thames and Hudson; 1988.

Spencer T. *The Iconography of Crabtree. The Crabtree Orations 1954–1994.* London, England: Crabtree Foundation; 1997.

Spolidorio MG, Labruna MB, Mantovani E, et al. Novel spotted fever rickettsiosis, Brazil. *Emerg Infect Dis.* 2010;16:521–523.

EMERGING
INFECTIOUS DISEASES®

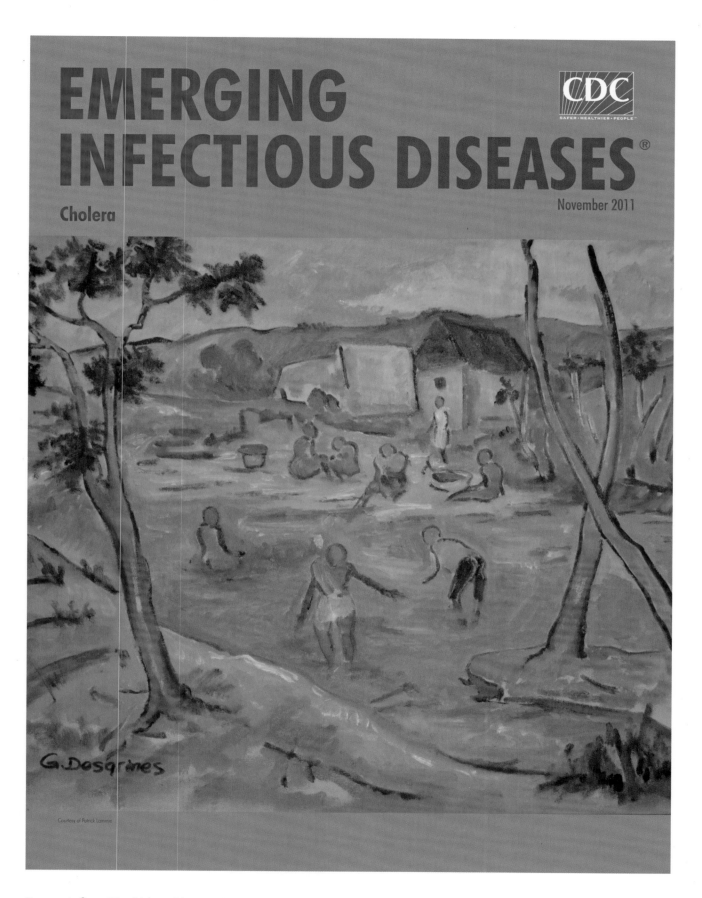

Cholera

November 2011

G. Desgrines

Courtesy of Patrick Lammie

PERSISTENCE OF MEMORY AND THE COMMA BACILLUS

"That anyone should condescend to die of cholera at the bidding of so insignificant a creature as the comma bacillus," wrote Marcel Proust, should not be astonishing to those in the know. Plagued by illness from childhood, the author was very much in tune with medicine, which he pondered often in *Remembrance of Things Past* (1913), his monumental novel on the nature of memory. He also knew about cholera. His father, eminent physician and public health pioneer Achille-Andrien Proust, dedicated much of his life to promoting *cordon sanitaire* for the control of the disease, convinced that "questions of international hygiene reach beyond the borders established by politics." The elder Proust's idea, ahead of his time, challenged free trade, so it was not until the Bombay cholera epidemic of 1877 that the concept of quarantine prevailed over commercialism and self-interest.

Marcel Proust was proud of his father. If visitors to the house were ever unwell, he was wont to ask them, "Would you like Papa to come to see you?" Once, when he made the offer to Anatole France, the man of letters replied, "My dear young friend, I should never dare to consult your father; I'm not important enough for him. The only patients he takes on nowadays are river basins!" Indeed, Dr. Proust had turned to public health. At great personal risk, he had cared for many a cholera patient during the 1866 epidemic in France and came to understand that individual treatment could not defeat this disease but prevention might control it. An early authority on epidemiology and a tireless advocate of an international sanitation system against disease spread, he is known in the history of medicine for his single-minded devotion to achieving the exclusion of cholera from the borders of Europe—this, some 20 years before Robert Koch identified the causative agent of the disease.

A severe infection spread by water contaminated with human waste, cholera was likely known in antiquity. Hippocrates and Galen described a compatible set of symptoms, and many sources point to similar illness, always present and frequently epidemic, in the plains of the Ganges River. In his landmark paper identifying the cause of the disease, Koch pinpointed the Ganges Delta as the *Heimat* (homeland) of cholera.

Many studied the scourge. In 1854, Filippo Pacini in Florence described vibrios in the intestinal contents of cholera victims and was amazed at their large numbers in the mucus and desquamated epithelial cells. He described the culprit as "an organic living substance of parasitic nature which can reproduce itself and thereby produce a specific disease." In London, John Snow demonstrated the role of water as carrier of the disease, prompting local authorities to, reluctantly, remove the handle of the notorious Broad Street pump. But it was not until 1884, during the outbreak in Egypt, when Koch noted that the disease was a specific gastrointestinal infection caused by a comma-shaped bacillus, which he isolated in the laboratory and named *Vibrio cholerae*. And it was not until 1965 that the Judicial Committee on Bacteriological Nomenclature ruled that the organism should be known as *Vibrio cholerae* Pacini 1854.

Cholera can strike anywhere when sanitary conditions are compromised and the causative agent is present. After a short incubation period of 2 or 3 days, the patient becomes ill with serious diarrhea and nausea followed, in severe cases, by extreme dehydration and death. Early European observers were struck by the patients' mummified appearance due to the draining of fluid from soft tissues.

Modern knowledge about cholera dates from the beginning of the 19th century, with seven major pandemics from 1800 to 1995, and has seen great progress in treatment if not prevention. With oral rehydration therapy, few patients should die if clean water is available. But floods and other natural disasters, along with social and economic ills favoring unsanitary conditions, compromise clean water supplies. Increased travel, population movements, and global conflict facilitate microbial traffic. Far from disappearing, cholera shows its ugly head as soon as the opportunity arises.

In October 2010, an outbreak of cholera was confirmed in Haiti. The two required conditions for emergence were present: *V. cholerae* introduced into the population and breaches in the water, sanitation, and hygiene infrastructure permitting exposure to contaminated water.

The Bathers, painted by Georges Desarmes, provides a glimpse of life on the Artibonite River and the bordering communities before the outbreak. Desarmes, born Yves Michaud in Port-au-Prince, began his artistic career working with Nehemy Jean, a well-traveled Haitian artist with diverse training in the United States and elsewhere. In the mid-1970s, Michaud met and went to work with Carlo Jean-Jacques, a Haitian impressionist; and in 2000, he started to paint in an entirely new style and assumed the name Georges Desarmes. Since then he has painted impressions of Haitian life.

In *The Bathers*, the artist captures the ease and communal charm of living along the river bank lined with tiny homes and populated with locals relating to each other on a personal level as they cool off. The scene is lyrical, spare, sunny, pre-cholera. On this day, this is the center of the universe, and this is the life. The artist captures the gist of it in a way only an impressionist could. As Proust would put it, "it's a country to be happy in." Yet this scene has since moved to another sphere, much like Proust's impressionist moments in time.

Refusing to recognize false boundaries, cholera encompasses the frailties of political conflict and the aftermath of mass travel and increased human contact. Since no outbreaks were seen in the Caribbean since the mid-19th century, it was said that Haiti had no memory of or experience in handling cholera. But Proust would disagree. The memory was there: Ships pull in harbors with unknown pestilent cargo. Sanitary conditions are not optimal. Contraband microbes hop off and settle in new areas among populations with no immunity or infrastructure to prevent rapid spread of disease.

Desarmes's lyrical impression of the waterfront meets *Remembrance of Things Past*. Proust struggled with the concept of involuntary memory, in which everyday cues evoke recollection of things past. But human history benefits more from voluntary memory, a deliberate effort to recall the past. Unless that happens, no one should be surprised if an inconsequential microbe causing a preventable and treatable disease continues to kill so many people.

Bibliography

Carter WC. *Marcel Proust: A Life*. New Haven, CT: Yale University Press; 2000.

Reimer AR, van Domselaar G, Stroika S, et al. Comparative genomics of *Vibrio cholerae* from Haiti, Asia, and Africa. *Emerg Infect Dis*. 2011;17:2113–2121.

Straus B. Achille-Adrien Proust, MD: doctor to river basins. *Bull N Y Acad Med*. 1974; 50:833–838.

Talkington D, Bopp C, Tarr C, et al. Characterization of toxigenic *Vibrio cholerae* from Haiti, 2010–2011. *Emerg Infect Dis*. 2011;17:2122–2129.

EMERGING
INFECTIOUS DISEASES®

A Peer-Reviewed Journal Tracking and Analyzing Disease Trends   Vol.9, No.2, February 2003

EID Online
www.cdc.gov/eid

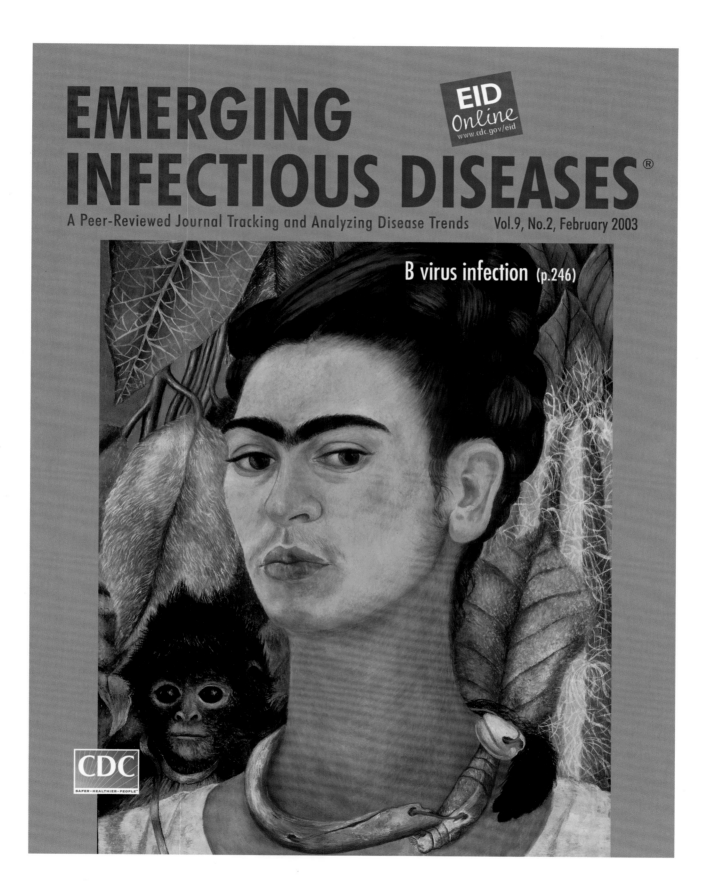

B virus infection (p.246)

CDC
SAFER·HEALTHIER·PEOPLE™

EXOTIC PETS AND ZOONOTIC PUZZLES

Frida Kahlo was born in Mexico City, the third daughter of a German father and a Spanish and Native American mother. Her life was marred by physical trauma—from childhood polio that left her with a limp, to serious injury in 1926, when a bus she was riding collided with a streetcar. Lifelong pain and its psychological aftermath had a profound effect on her artistic development.

Kahlo was well educated and fiercely independent. A frail girl with a limp, she set out to be a tomboy, an intellectual, a heartbreaker, and a communist. Relentless physical pain, marital strife, and emotional rejection marked the course of her life. Her work, which incorporates Mexican folk motifs and particularly the small votive pictures known as *retablos*, exudes powerful feeling and is unlike that of any of her contemporary Mexican muralists. Characterized by boundless energy and strength, her paintings represent her passion for meaning and truth, her feistiness and defiance of limits, her intimate acquaintance with suffering, and finally her poignant acknowledgment of things as they are.

Kahlo's artistic talent was recognized by the French poet and critic André Breton in 1938, when he visited Mexico. Breton, who had studied medicine and worked on psychiatric wards during World War I, was a founder and chief promoter of the surrealist movement. The movement, partly borne of post–World War disillusionment, promoted a "revolution of the mind" against a civilization that seemed to be lowering human aspirations and proliferating human misery. Surrealism sought to synthesize humans and their world, eliminating the barriers between dream and reality, reason and madness, persons and things.

During her early association with Breton in Mexico, which he termed a "naturally surrealist country," Kahlo worked alongside the surrealists, yet she denied any connection with them: "They thought I was a surrealist . . . but I wasn't. I never painted dreams, I painted my own reality." Even if she never espoused surrealist ideology, Kahlo seemed to embody it. She transcended her physical suffering and delved into untapped emotional depths for universal truth, which she uncovered and brought to the viewer in raw, brilliant color. In a surrealist manner, Kahlo's work was permeated by her tempestuous life and cannot be fully understood apart from it.

From her vivid *Self-Portrait*, Frida Kahlo casts a pensive but challenging look at a world that denied her the comforts of health. Like an exotic flower, she embellishes the luscious tropical tableau. Yet, in spite of her regal demeanor and the scene's vibrant hues, something is troubling about the picture. Menace lurks in nature itself, which though seemingly embracing, is not unqualifiedly benign. The enigmatic presence of the monkey heightens the portrait's uneasiness. Might it be the devil, as purported in Kahlo's native Mexico?

Nonhuman primates are frequent human playmates in the arts, the circus, and the streets—always amusing, romantic, and mysterious, and sometimes dark. Might the monkey on Kahlo's back be the harbinger of ill health? Like her contemporaries, Kahlo knew little of her close phylogenetic kinship with her pet or the extreme caution prescribed by this kinship. The threat signaled by the presence of a primate, be it turbulence in Kahlo's life or herpes B viruses in ours, remains uncharted. The monkey on our back is to decipher the zoonotic puzzle of infection that perpetuates suffering and limits the immense capacity of the human spirit.

Bibliography

André Breton (1896–1966). Available at: http://www.kirjasto.sci.fi/abreton.htm. Accessed December 18, 2002.

Lucie-Smith E. *Lives of the Great 20th Century Artists*. London, England: Thames and Hudson; 1999.

EMERGING INFECTIOUS DISEASES®

October 2012

Human–Primate Encounters

HUMAN MINUS THREE PIECES OF HAIR

At age 61, Mori Sosen changed the first character of his name to one meaning "monkey." So close had he become to the subject of his paintings. To learn how to paint the animals convincingly, he lived for a time in the mountains, their natural environment, not relying as others before him on copying their images from Chinese art. His mastery in depicting the Japanese macaque earned him the title "undisputed master" from Dutch Orientalist Robert van Gulik (1910–1967). In his book, *The Gibbon in China*, van Gulik translated Confucian scholar Kimura Kenkadō's account of the animal's arrival in Japan. "In the winter of the sixth year of the era (1809), a gibbon was shown in Osaka. . . . Although we have heard the word 'gibbon' since olden times and seen pictures of him, we never had seen a live specimen, and therefore a large crowd assembled to see this gibbon. Generally he resembled a large macaque, and figure and fur are very similar." Mori Sosen created a graphic record of this sensational event.

Not much is known about his life but that he grew up with and around artists, started his training with his father Mori Jokansai, and lived most of his life in Osaka. Mori Sosen's legacy is his painting of animals, particularly monkeys, their personalities and attitudes as well as their coats and the movement of their muscles underneath. So well did he depict the nature of monkeys that he was accused of being their descendent. He established, with his brother Shūhō, a school of animal painting along the lines of the *Maruyama-Shijō* school in Kyoto. Shūhō's son studied there under Maruyama Ōkyo, an expert in a style influenced by Western realism and direct observation. The *Shijō* school promoted synthesizing this modern development with the local trend toward the decorative and stylized.

Monkey Performing the Sanbasō Dance showcases both Mori Sosen's favorite subject matter and his artistic style, a blend of realism and expressiveness. The action is set against a vacant background, the viewer drawn toward the main figure. Bold deliberate strokes outline the facial features, right hand and both feet of the animal, and folds in the kimono. Smudged strokes from a dry brush draw the ruffled texture of the fur against the black cap and smooth, mostly unpainted surface of the clothing. The monkey, mouth pursed with concentration, eyes fixed on some point outside the painting, holds a fan in one hand, and with the other, it raises a cluster of bells. The right leg is lifted in a dance step, while the left, toes curled inward for better balance, is rigid. During the Edo period (1603–1868), Kabuki theater programs began at dawn with a dance. In the final of three scenes in this dance, "the bell-tree," the dancer would shake a wand covered with small bells. Along these lines, the monkey in Mori Sosen's work lifts the bells in performing the Sanbasō, a dance celebrating the New Year, the first day of the Monkey Year.

Macaques, more than 20 species of *Macaca*, a genus of Old World monkeys mostly found in Asia, occupy a geographic range second only to that of humans in its extent. Their habitat varies from near desert to rainforest, from sea level to snow-covered mountain tops. The Japanese macaque, also known as snow monkey, which has been reported at an elevation of 3,180 m, representing the northernmost nonhuman primate population in the world, has gained some notoriety for visiting a hot spring in Nagano to find comfort from the cold in winter.

Culturally, this monkey has been a metaphor, a polysemic symbol throughout Japanese history—now a mediator between gods and humans, now a scapegoat, now a clown. Because of its unique role as similar to, yet different from, humans, the Japanese macaque was used to define what it means to be human and alternatively what it means to be a monkey: "human minus three pieces of hair," to the Japanese. This definition satisfied both the affinity between humans and monkeys and the animal's local status just below grade.

The monkey's role as mediator between gods and humans was long lived and well established. It implied possession of supernatural powers, which were often expressed in ritual dances with music. The monkey was believed a guardian that could cure disease in horses and secure good crops as mediator between the Mountain Deity and humans. This status diminished gradually. The monkey was secularized and demoted, becoming the object of ridicule, a scapegoat, for lacking (even if only by three pieces of hair) the essence of humanness. Though a monkey dance performance still likely showcases human superiority, the powerful metaphorical presence persists, despite the animal's virtual disappearance from everyday human contact outside the zoo.

Around the world, the status of macaques and their connection with humans continues to evolve. The Japanese tradition that the monkey was a scapegoat for a human victim of smallpox or of another disease, which persisted for centuries, is no longer held. In more recent times the animals have served instead as models for human disease, providing through their own infections or experimental studies, insight into pathogenic mechanisms, treatments, and vaccine approaches for human infectious agents, among them, hepatitis B, influenza virus, flaviviruses, and *Plasmodium* spp. Some infections (HIV-2, *P. knowlesii*) have been transmitted from nonhuman primates to humans, suggesting that the role of these primates as "mediators" persists, but some, including measles and tuberculosis, can go both ways, with infected humans compromising the health of nonhuman primate. Because of the infections in the monkeys, an employee health vaccination program was launched, potentially preventing tetanus among workers.

In one study, a colony of Japanese macaques saw a mass die-off attributed to severe soil contamination by *Clostridium tetani* in the facility maintaining the animals. In China, *Cryptosporidium* spp., *Giardia duodenalis*, and *Enterocytozoon bieneusi* organisms were detected in free-range rhesus monkeys in a popular public park. Most genotypes and subtypes detected were anthroponotic, which indicates that these animals, after becoming infected from exposure to infected humans, may have become reservoirs for human cryptosporidiosis, giardiasis, and microsporidiosis. In Afghanistan, bites from macaques may have exposed US troops and presumably the Afghanis to serious infections, among them rabies, B virus, and tetanus. In Africa, nonhuman primates may be acting as a zoonotic reservoir of *P. vivax* in regions where the human population is almost entirely refractory. If so, with human encroachment into nonhuman primate habitats, the chances of susceptible humans encountering the parasite will increase.

As it lifts up the bells to ring in the New Year 1800, Mori Sosen's beloved monkey in the flawless kimono continues the age-old dance celebrating our phylogenetic closeness. Because of this closeness, humans and nonhuman primates are susceptible to many of the same infections, minus three pieces of hair or not.

Bibliography

Culleton RL, Mendes PE. Duffy phenotype and Plasmodium vivax infections in humans and apes, Africa. *Emerg Infect Dis.* 2012;18:1704–1705.

Gardner MB, Luciw PA. Macaque models of human infectious disease. *ILAR J.* 2008;49: 220–255.

Mease LE, Baker KA. Monkey bites among US military members, Afghanistan, 2011. *Emerg Infect Dis.* 2012;18:1647–1649.

Nakano T, Nakamura S, Yamamoto A, et al. Tetanus as cause of mass die-off of captive Japanese macaques, Japan, 2008. *Emerg Infect Dis.* 2012;18:1633–1635.

Ohnuki-Tierney E. The monkey as self in Japanese culture. In: Ohnuki-Tierney E., ed. *Culture Through Time.* Palo Alto, CA: Stanford University Press; 1991:128–153.

Pacific Asia Museum. Nature of the beast. Available at: http://www.pacificasiamuseum.org/japanesepaintings/html/essay2.stm. Accessed June 26, 2012.

Poster AG. *Japanese Paintings of the Shijō School.* New York, NY: The Brooklyn Museum; 1981.

Smith L, Harris V, Clark T. *Japanese Art: Masterpieces in the British Museum.* London, England: The British Museum Press; 1990.

van Gulik RH. *The Gibbon in China. An essay in Chinese Animal Lore.* Leiden, The Netherlands: EJ Brill; 1967.

Ye J, Xiao L, Ma J, et al. Anthroponotic enteric parasites in monkeys in public park, China. *Emerg Infect Dis.* 2012;18:1640–1643.

Vol 18, No 6, June 2012

EMERGING
INFECTIOUS DISEASES®

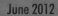

June 2012

Prion Diseases

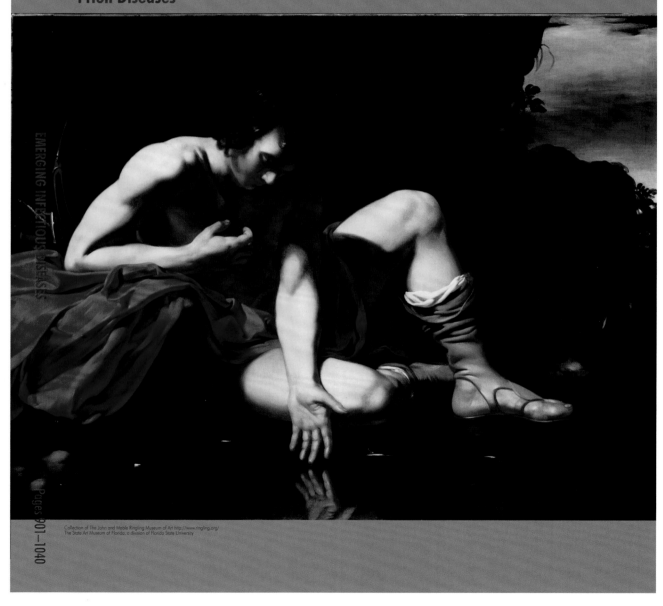

Pages 901–1040

I RHYME /TO SEE MYSELF, TO SET THE DARKNESS ECHOING[2]

"As a child, they could not keep me from wells," wrote Seamus Heaney in his version of the Narcissus myth. "I loved the dark drop, the trapped sky, the smells / of waterweed, fungus and dank moss." In countless versions, the ancient myth strikes a universal chord: person sees self, meets death. Ovid told of handsome Narcissus and Echo, the nymph who fell in love when she saw him "chasing frightened deer into his nets." Rejected, she wasted away, until nothing was left but her voice, "heard by all." He, "Tired from both his enthusiasm for hunting and from the heat," rested a spell, caught glimpse of his reflection in a pool of water, and fell in love with "all the things for which he himself is admired." Unable to tear himself from the fateful reflection, he too wasted away. At this spot later sprouted narcissus, the flower.

Favored by poet and artist alike, the story intrigues anyone who searches for or reconstructs the self. In art, variations abound, among them one by the great Michelangelo Merisi da Caravaggio (1571–1610). Contrary to the conventions of his age, he painted directly from posed models, a practice that cultivated a new relationship between painting and viewer by promoting art not as fiction but as an extension of everyday experience, the physical content enriched with psychological tension. Gerard van Kuijl, Dutch painter and follower of Caravaggio, might have seen the master's *Narcissus* (1597) when he lived in Rome from 1629 to 1631.

In the 17th century, many artists from the northern Low Countries worked abroad or were influenced by others who had traveled and returned, bringing new styles to the local market. Their work strayed from the polders, woods, and dunes of the Dutch Golden Age to the biblical and secular, with human figures dominating the canvas. These artists exerted a lasting influence by introducing one of the main currents of baroque art into the Netherlands. The Caravaggists were mainly artists from Utrecht, who visited Italy and worked in the style of Caravaggio, characterized by realist drama and strong interplay of light and dark. This style also prevailed outside Utrecht, affecting Rembrandt and his followers.

In van Kuijl's *Narcissus*, expert shading betrays Caravaggist influence as do the baroque shapes and style. In both the Caravaggio and van Kuijl renditions, the figure is wrapped in a mystical, isolating, introspective dark. But, despite the striking similarities, van Kuijl's approach is individualized. While Caravaggio moved the figure into his own times, showing no traces of classical attire, van Kuijl maintained topical decorum and a trace of the pastoral. Overall, it seems as if the two images represented a sequence. In the earlier painting the figure is actively engaged with his reflection, almost interactive, agile, embracing. In van Kuijl's work, having given into the overwhelming attraction, the figure is entranced, dreamy, stochastic.

---

2 From "Personal Helicon" by Seamus Heaney, available at www.ibiblio.org/ipa/poems/heaney/personal_helicon.php

The theme of Narcissus is not new to science, having been exhaustively addressed in psychoanalysis and come down to us as narcissism and the narcissistic personality. In one iteration, the theme overlaps with the ever-popular myth of Pygmalion, the sculptor in antiquity, who fell in love not with his image but with his work—a female statue he created, one so perfect that it was, in his estimation, more beautiful than any woman could ever be.

Breathing life into or animating a work of art was not the domain of Pygmalion alone. Lyric poet Pindar in his seventh "Olympic Ode" wrote, "The animated figures stand / Adorning every public street / And seem to breathe in stone, or move their marble / feet." Daedalus used to install voice in his statues, and Hephaestus created automata for his workshop. But these mechanical attempts with lifeless objects pale before more recent achievements, no less in modern medicine, which breathe life into dying human bodies with grafts, transfusions, and transplants, extending their tenure and the resilience of the species.

"Man," wrote Johann Wolfgang von Goethe in his novel *Elective Affinities*, "is a true Narcissus. He makes the whole world his mirror." The philosopher's interest was literary, an opportunity to unravel personal and social processes and interpret the meaning of human actions and events. He thought that, like the young Seamus Heaney, man could not pass up an opportunity "To stare, big-eyed Narcissus, into some spring." Nevertheless, as an adult, the poet himself found his early fascination with the well undignified. "I rhyme," he professed, "To see myself, to set the darkness echoing."

Goethe had no way of knowing that the time would come when humans would literally be able to re-create that which so fascinated them as myth and metaphor—not only re-create their image in a poem or, like Pygmalion, in art but also in the flesh. For loving one's creation is certainly easy to fall into, even in science. A more resilient human with healthier and longer lasting parts is the reflection we look for in the well, a reflection too of improved medical knowledge, expertise, and technology: properly used antimicrobial drugs; preventive screening; and growth hormone and dura mater grafts from cadavers, the bold modern equivalent of magic and automata in statues. Yet the echo we expect to hear from the darkness is often interrupted by emerging pathogens and often, unawares, by ourselves.

The history of medicine is filled with examples of unintended consequences. A concern since the time of Hippocrates, "to do no harm" is a continuing chapter with an abundance of contemporary examples. Reliance on a single class of antimicrobial drugs for treatment of some infections heightens our vulnerability to emergence of resistance, requiring more treatment options. Preoperatively acquired emerging pathogens complicate liver transplantation, a problem threatening to increase, despite adequate infection control measures. On the other hand, comprehensive current tallies of global incidence of iatrogenic Creutzfeldt-Jakob disease identified no new sources of disease, indicating that current practices should continue to minimize the risk until blood screening is validated for human use and suggesting that, despite setbacks that make that glimpse of perfect self fatal, science diligently applied can still set the darkness echoing.

Bibliography

Bert F, Larroque B, Paugam-Burtz C, et al. Pretransplant fecal carriage of extended-spectrum β-lactamase–producing *Enterobacteriaceae* and infection after liver transplant, France. *Emerg Infect Dis.* 2012;18:908–916.

Brown P, Brandel J-P, Sato T, et al. Iatrogenic Creutzfeldt-Jakob disease: final assessment. *Emerg Infect Dis.* 2012;18:901–907.

Christiansen K. Caravaggio (Michelangelo Merisi) (1571–1610) and his followers. In: *Heilbrunn Timeline of Art History.* New York: The Metropolitan Museum of Art; 2000.

Kirkcaldy RD, Augostini P, Asbel LE, et al. *Trichomonas vaginalis* antimicrobial drug resistance in 6 US cities, STD Surveillance Network, 2009–2010. *Emerg Infect Dis.* 2012;18:939–943.

Ovid. *Metamorphoses.* Melville AD, trans. Oxford, England: Oxford University Press; 1986.

Pindar. The seventh Olympic ode. Available at: http://www.ebooksread.com/authors-eng/pindar/pindar-hci/page-3-pindar-hci.shtml. Accessed April 5, 2012.

Vol 13, No 5, May 2007

DEPARTMENT OF
HEALTH & HUMAN SERVICES
Public Health Service
Center for Disease Control and Prevention (CDC)
Atlanta, GA 30333

Official Business
Penalty for Private Use $300

Return Service Requested

EMERGING INFECTIOUS DISEASES

Pages 681-814

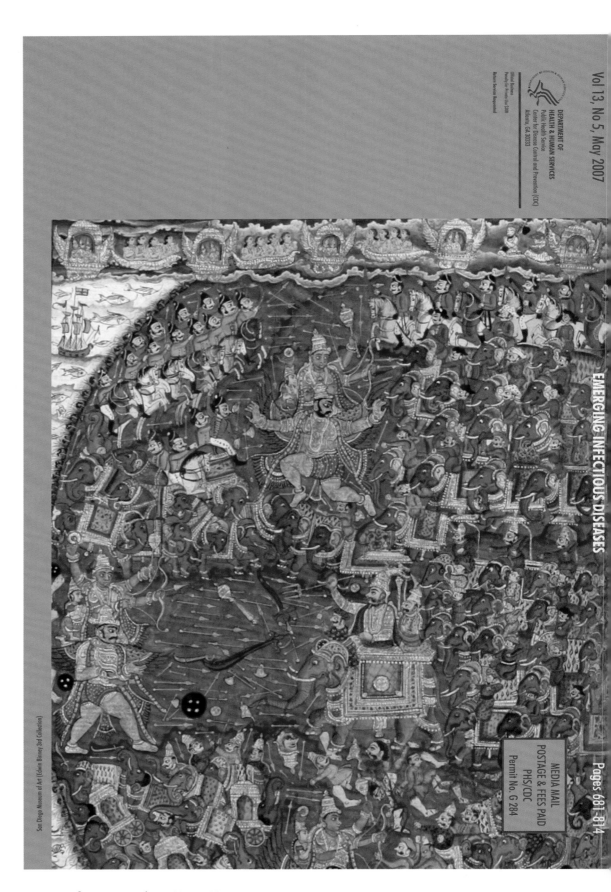

San Diego Museum of Art (Edwin Binney 3rd Collection)

MERGING
NFECTIOUS DISEASES

May 2007

ntimicrobial Resistance

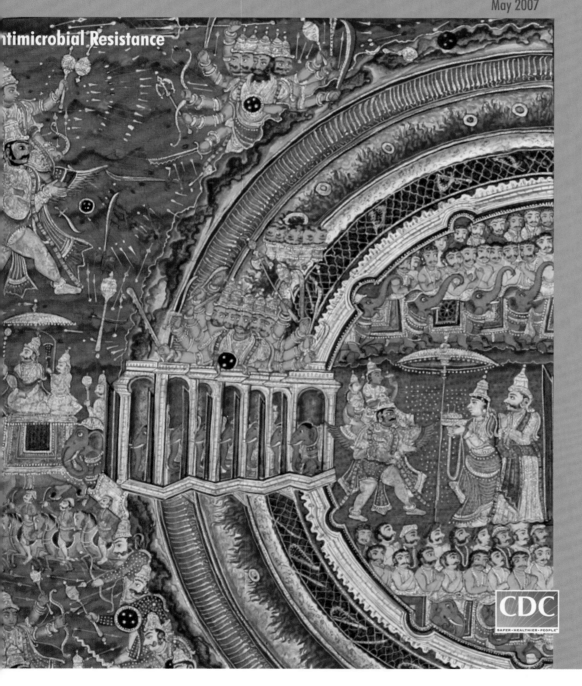

CDC
SAFER · HEALTHIER · PEOPLE

PROTECT ME, LORD, FROM OIL, FROM WATER, FROM FIRE, AND FROM ANTS AND SAVE ME FROM FALLING INTO THE HANDS OF FOOLS[3]

Indian paintings on paper, known as "miniatures," can be found in books from as far back as the 11th century, most from the 14th through the 19th century. They vary from postage stamp size to more than a yard in height and are called miniatures partly to distinguish them from murals, which they followed as a genre. Like the good books they inhabited, they were portable and intimate, meant to be appreciated from close up and, duly treasured, they were tucked away to be handled only from time to time, with care.

Miniature paintings were collaborative, created by groups of artists specialized in drawing, portraiture, background, or border illustration and were exclusively commissioned by patrons—princes, merchants, religious leaders. The importance attached to patronage can be traced in the colophons of surviving books. We know virtually nothing about the anonymous artist who created the painting but can often trace at whose "lotus feet" it was placed when completed.

Though "All the blessings of heaven" were bestowed on the patron of a manuscript or series, great patrons did not emerge until the late 15th century. Soon after, during the Mughal Empire, interest in art peaked, along with patronage, and schools of painting developed and flourished.

Miniatures were often painted on a wash: sheets of paper glued together and laminated. Ground white chalk or lead formed the foundation for layers of transparent watercolor in vivid, exotic pigments, from gum arabic or crushed seeds of the tamarind. Indian yellow was made of dried urine from cows fed on mango leaves. Gold, in leaf or liquid, embellished clothing and jewelry. Detail was created laboriously with fine brushes of hair from live squirrels, luster achieved from burnishing the surface, which also bonded pigment layers to the support. Book pages were intricately illustrated, some double-sided, with calligraphic elements on the verso.

The folio on this month's cover comes from the *Bhagavata Purana*, a celebrated text in Hindu sacred literature recited daily by millions. Though favored and revered by painters and patrons, the *Purana*, with its collection of "ancient and wondrous tales of the Lord" Krishna, has rarely been illustrated with such exuberance. The embroidered cover of this manuscript, which contains 217 paintings, identifies it as volume 6 in a series. It was written on European paper. A seal on the flyleaf reads, "His Highness, Rajah of Mysore."

Eyes are naturally drawn to Krishna. His name literally means "black" or "dark" or "all-attractive," and he has a very distinct iconography. In his countless avatars, from Vishnu to simple human, his beauty is irresistible, his complexion "tinged with the hue of blue clouds." Clad in golden silk, he rides the sun-bird Garuda. The philosophy of this God/cowherd is captured in the epic of the Hindu faith, the *Bhagavad-Gita*.

---

3 Prayer "uttered by a manuscript." Found at the end of medieval Indian texts.

Krishna Storms the Citadel of Naraka recounts the God's exploits against a demon king, a menace who commits atrocities, even against his own mother, the Earth Goddess. Aboard Garuda with his consort Satyabhama, Krishna wings his way to the demon's citadel, "Which heart would not quail at the loud blast . . . from the Lord's conch?" The enemy is barricaded in his impregnable island city, inaccessible by "hilly fortifications and mounted missiles and weaponry" and unapproachable with "moats of water and fire and belts of stormy winds."

Krishna, in true form, is Vishnu, four-armed and impervious to "thousands of fearful and strong snares." He faces Mura, the five-headed demon (upper right), who soon falls, "like a mountain summit struck by a thunderbolt." Mura's seven sons move in, advancing, "discharging volleys of shafts, swords, maces, darts, double-edged swords and javelins" to perish, too, along with their armies. Naraka joins in and succumbs to Krishna, who appears everywhere, "like a cloud emblazoned in a streak of lightning." The citadel is penetrated. Inside, the Earth Goddess, bowing, offers Krishna "a pair of earrings resplendent with jewels and chased in the purest gold . . . a garland of forest flowers, the umbrella of Varuna."

The unfolding spectacle encompasses the heavens, engaging with ease gods, humans, animals, and mythologic beasts. Tiny figures move about purposefully, elephants carry on with dignity, seas are alive with fish. The monumental story is painted with assurance, as if it could have happened only in this orderly and brilliant way. And flying arrows and severed heads notwithstanding, the event seems a pageant, the celebration of a shift in the balance of power, an interaction whose outcome was never in doubt.

The citadel of Naraka with its formidable fortifications and hordes of defenders begs an equivalent in the microbial world. And not only because vermin threaten everything, even books. In the eternal, complicated interactions between microbes and hosts, supremacy and survival are closely knit. Host defenses are inevitably overcome by adaptation and change, until more sophisticated, specialized defenses can be built. Microbes develop resistance. Hosts mount additional defense. Microbes regroup and reappear in manifestations and avatars rivaling those of Krishna himself.

Bibliography

Bhaktivedanta VedaBase Network. Sri Brahma-samhita: Chapter 5 verse 30. Available at: http://www.vedabase.net/bs/5/30/en1. Accessed March 14, 2007.

Goswamy BN, Smith C. *Domains of Wonder: Selected Masterworks of Indian Painting.* Frome, England: Butler and Tanner; 2005.

National Gallery of Australia. A stream of stories: Indian miniatures; http://www.nga.gov.au/ Conservation/Paper/IndianMiniatures.html; accessed March 23, 2007.

Prabhavananda S, Isherwood C, trans. *The Song of God: Bhagavad-Gita.* London, England: Phoenix House; 1964.

EMERGING
INFECTIOUS DISEASES

EID Online www.cdc.gov/eid

A Peer-Reviewed Journal Tracking and Analyzing Disease Trends

Vol.10, No.5, May 2004

The SARS Patient

CDC
SAFER·HEALTHIER·PEOPLE

THE SARS PATIENT

"Goya in gratitude to his friend Arrieta for the skill and care with which he saved his life in his acute and dangerous illness suffered at the end of the year 1819 at the age of 73. He painted it in 1820," reads the inscription at the bottom of Goya's *Self-Portrait.* An affirmation of medical practice, the painting is also an acknowledgment of human compassion, a quality the artist thought extremely rare.

Conflicted in his acceptance of the world and in his portrayal of it and deeply mistrustful of human nature, Goya lingered on the dark side as he painted the full spectrum of life experiences. During his long artistic career, he dwelled on the tensions of Spanish society of his day, whose institutions, including medicine, he gleefully satirized (*Of What Illness Will He Die?* [1799]).

Deaths in his family and debilitating illness throughout his years often interfered with his work and left him weak and disillusioned. "Neither sight, nor pen nor inkwell; all these I lack and all that is plentiful is my will," the painter remarked to a friend regarding his loss of hearing, poor health, and frail disposition. Near the end of his life, once again he became seriously ill. Overcoming his natural aversion to authority, he entrusted himself to the care of a physician friend. When the health crisis subsided, Goya created *Self-Portrait with Doctor Arrieta.*

Unlike most paintings of his later years, which evoke horror and darkness, this double portrait imprints a gentle aspect of humanity on the mild physiognomies of physician and patient. Even so, rather than a departure from his sinister worldview, the painting of one man tending to another was a gesture of gratitude after deliverance from death.

The portrait is an empathetic rendition not of Goya alone but of the universal human patient. Isolated but for the intruding shadows witnessing his pending demise, in a drab dressing gown, generic, exposed, and vulnerable, Goya embodies the plight of the sick. Withered and limp, unkempt and undignified, he is reduced to an infantile state, to be comforted and cajoled, humored with therapeutic potions and measures, and ordered to obey.

Gone is the thundering presence, the compelling personality, the artistic genius, the signature mistrust of human nature. Opinions and attitudes were shed at the sickroom door, along with his everyday clothes and his ability to walk and control his life. With his private condition on public display, he is at the mercy of his caretakers. Clutching the carmine blanket between him and the world, he succumbs to the physician's sympathetic embrace and, near death, sinks deeper into isolation.

The kindly physician is warm and obliging, if not unduly hopeful. Aware of his limited capacity to reverse the course of illness, he focuses on what is within his capacity: comfort and support. He draws near the patient, as if to become one with him and propel his own strength and energy onto the ailing body. The closeness of his embrace equals his instinct to alleviate pain and his oblivion of risk to himself from proximity to the patient. As he firmly administers the medication, his face wears the look of the stoic philosopher and the eagerness of the medical intern.

An astute observer of the human condition, Goya understood the tragic nature of disease, often manifested in our inability to prevent its onset, control its course, and predict its outcome. Understanding of infection has burgeoned since 1820, yet patient isolation, vulnerability, uncertainty, and untimely death remain unresolved. In emerging disease puzzles, where treatment is sometimes administered while large pieces are still being assembled, the old measures of infection control and quarantine are challenged by new environmental, social, and scientific developments. Contagion, unknown to Dr. Arrieta, is particularly pertinent in diseases like SARS, where the threat is not fully quantified until, unlike the images in Goya's double portrait, the patient and the caretaker are one.

Bibliography

Lau JTF. SARS transmission, risk factors, and prevention in Hong Kong. *Emerg Infect Dis.* 2004;10:587–592.

Matilla JM. *Goya*. Madrid, Spain: TF Arts Gráficas; 2000.

Sylvester D. *About Modern Art*. New Haven, CT: Yale University Press; 2001.

Technology, Industry, Travel, and Commerce

"Three tribes of Babylonians," Herodotus wrote, "eat nothing but fish, which they catch and dry in the sun. They pound the dried fish in a mortar with a pestle and sift through a cloth then mix with liquid and bake like bread." Such are their customs, he reported, "Having no physicians, they bring the sick to the agora to receive advice from passers-by who have similar ailments."

Travel anecdotes fill Herodotus' histories. He recorded them so that "happenings will not be lost to human memory nor great and fantastic deeds . . . fade." Mocked for his accounts of outlandish behavior, Herodotus got no respect until centuries later, when similar unlikely behavior was seen elsewhere, and its anthropological and ethnographic roots were verified. Human fascination with travel to mysterious lands has occupied artists as well as writers throughout the ages. Henri Matisse's *Icarus*, a work used on a cover of *Emerging Infectious Diseases*, memorializes the quintessential human desire to explore the world, even when the circumstances are not ideal. Australian painter Cameron Hayes (b. 1969), whose work oddly named *The Russians knew perfectly well that the happiness of the African animals was that they had such low expectations—before the pets were introduced* appeared on a cover of *Emerging Infectious Diseases*, offered his own narrative version of travel.

Hayes's interest in human behavior is reflected in all his work. He traces his roots far from today's art centers, even if he exhibits in galleries all over the world. Born in Sydney and now based in Melbourne, he has explored the effects of European settlement on the Aboriginal population in Milikapiti on Melville Island off the northern coast of Australia. He has articulated in his art the loss of cultural identity and health to often well-intentioned outside influences. This journey inward sharpened his vision of today's global scene, which he views with suspicion and satirizes without mercy in his paintings.

Travel is a potent force in the emergence of disease. Migration of humans has been the pathway for disseminating infection throughout recorded history and will likely continue to shape its emergence, frequency, and spread in geographic areas and populations. When they travel, humans carry with them their genetic makeup, past infections, culture, customs, and behavior. Microbes, animals, plants, and other biological elements also accompany them. Today's massive movement of humans and materials sets the stage for mixing diverse genetic pools at unprecedented rates and combinations. Concomitant changes in the environment, climate, technology, land use, human behavior, and demographics converge to favor the emergence of infectious diseases caused by a broad range of microbes in humans, as well as in plants and animals. Liubov Popova's *The Traveler* draws an eloquent connection between radical art movements, known as Russian avant-garde, and the explosion of travel around the world.

High-volume rapid movement characterizes not only travel but also other industries in modern society. In operations, including food production, that process or use products of biological origin, modern methods yield increased efficiency and reduced costs but can increase the chances of accidental contamination and amplify its effects. Globalization allows the introduction of agents from far away. A pathogen present in some raw material may find its way into a large batch of final product, as happened with the contamination of ground beef by *E. coli* strains causing hemolytic uremic syndrome. In the United States, the implicated *E. coli* strains generally are serotype O157:H7; other serotypes are more prominent in other countries. Diego Velázquez's *Old Woman Cooking Eggs* creates a bold contrast between food preparation then and now and invites speculation on the scarcity of food, common in the painter's time, and the food safety issues of today.

"Mad cow" disease, which emerged in Britain, possibly as an interspecies transfer of scrapie from sheep to cattle, may have happened because of changes in rendering processes. These changes may have allowed incompletely inactivated prion proteins that contaminate sheep byproducts to be fed to cattle. The disease wreaked havoc on the livestock industry in the United Kingdom, causing the death of 200,000 cattle. Nearly 4.5 million asymptomatic cattle were slaughtered as a preventive measure. Through trade, the disease was exported around the globe. *Moschophoros (Calf-Bearer)*, attributed to Phaidimos, exemplifies the ancient symbiotic relationship between humans and animals at the same time testifying to the shortcomings of that relationship manifested in animal sacrifices then and now. As a possible solution to this ancient dilemma, American epidemiologist Calvin Schwabe proposed in the 1980s a unified approached against zoonotic diseases. This approach, "one medicine," is discussed in the context of Edward Hicks's *Peaceable Kingdom*.

SARS, an emerging disease still without cure, has demonstrated how easily health care systems can be overwhelmed by the demands for patient screening and care, particularly with the special infection control requirements that come with a respiratory illness of this kind. Similarly, it posed troubling questions about how and when travel and commerce should be constrained in the context of communicable disease. SARS spread was eventually contained by quarantine and strict infection control in hospitals but not before it had traveled from the Far East to Toronto. Vincent van Gogh's *The Prison Courtyard* links the angst and isolation of the troubled painter with the physical and emotional isolation of SARS patients, many of them frontline health care providers.

Infectious diseases emerge as a result of changes in technology and industry. Such advances in medicine as blood transfusions and human-to-human and animal-to-human organ and tissue transplants create new pathways for the spread of certain infections. Health care environments are fertile grounds for disease emergence not only because they are filled with patients but also because the medical devices used for treatment can become vehicles of pathogen transmission.

The syringe and needle have been called the most effective medical vector of infectious disease, particularly for their big role in the transmission of HIV. Francisco Roa's *Sands Flowers* offers the opportunity for discussing the unending cycle of old and new diseases. The painter sought answers in the power of exacting detail, an approach also used in science, where answers sometimes also lie in improved technology, better medicines, vaccines, and diagnostic tests.

"They bury their Dead with their Heads directly downwards; because they hold an Opinion, that in eleven Thousand Moons they are all to rise again; in which Period, the Earth (which they conceive to be flat) will turn upside down, and by this Means they shall, at their Resurrection, be found ready standing on their Feet," wrote Jonathan Swift about the inhabitants of Lilliput, in *Gulliver's Travels*. Swift, continuing in the tradition of Herodotus, wrote about travel adventures. But, an inveterate satirist, he spiced them liberally with biting wit intended to upset and reform a malfunctioning society. "The chief end I propose to myself in all my labours is to vex the world rather than divert it."

Human behavior, in ancient Babylon, Lilliput, or Milikapiti, has cultural, economic, and public health consequences. Ecotourism has attracted people to remote animal habitats, and commerce has moved animals to new environments. Despite evidence of disease risks, demand for exotic pets is high. Despite inherent hazards (Buruli ulcer, malaria, dengue, avian flu, norovirus infection), humans move freely around the globe. "People," Hayes says, "invariably find creative and elaborate ways of maintaining their perception, against all the available evidence, rather than questioning their perception of reality."

Bibliography

Cameron Hayes. Available at: http://www.feldmangallery.com/pages/artistsrffa/arthay01.html. Accessed October 24, 2008.

Herodotou musai. Athens, Greece: N. Michalopoulos; 1883.

The land of Cockaygne. Available at: http://www.soton.ac.uk/~wpwt/trans/cockaygn/coctrans.htm. Accessed November 13, 2008.

Potter P. Traveling light and the tyranny of higher expectations. Available at: http://wwwnc.cdc.gov/eid/article/15/1/ac-1501_article.htm. Accessed May 22, 2013.

Swift J. *Gulliver's Travels.* Norwalk, CT: The Heritage Press; 1968.

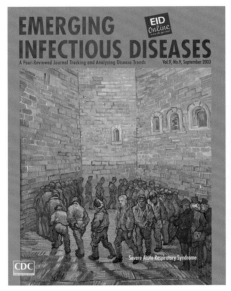

Severe Acute Respiratory Syndrome; http://dx.doi.org/10.3201/eid0909.AC0909

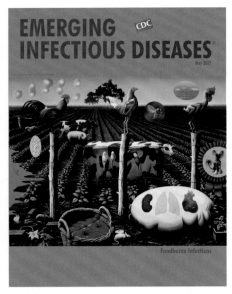

Foodborne Infections; http://dx.doi.org/10.3201/eid1505.AC1505

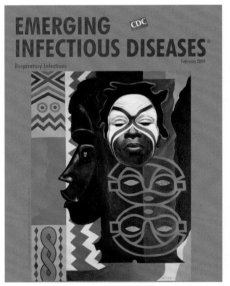

Respiratory Infections; http://dx.doi.org/10.3201/eid1502.AC1502

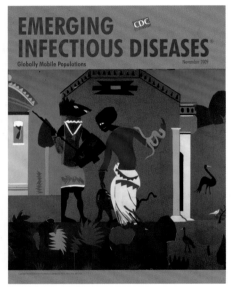

Globally Mobile Populations; http://dx.doi.org/10.3201/eid1511.AC1511

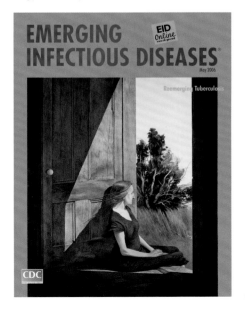

Reemergence of Tuberculosis; http://dx.doi.org/10.3201/eid1205.AC1205

EMERGING
INFECTIOUS DISEASES

EID Online
www.cdc.gov/eid

A Peer-Reviewed Journal Tracking and Analyzing Disease Trends

Vol.9, No.5, May 2003

Hazards of Travel (pg.525)

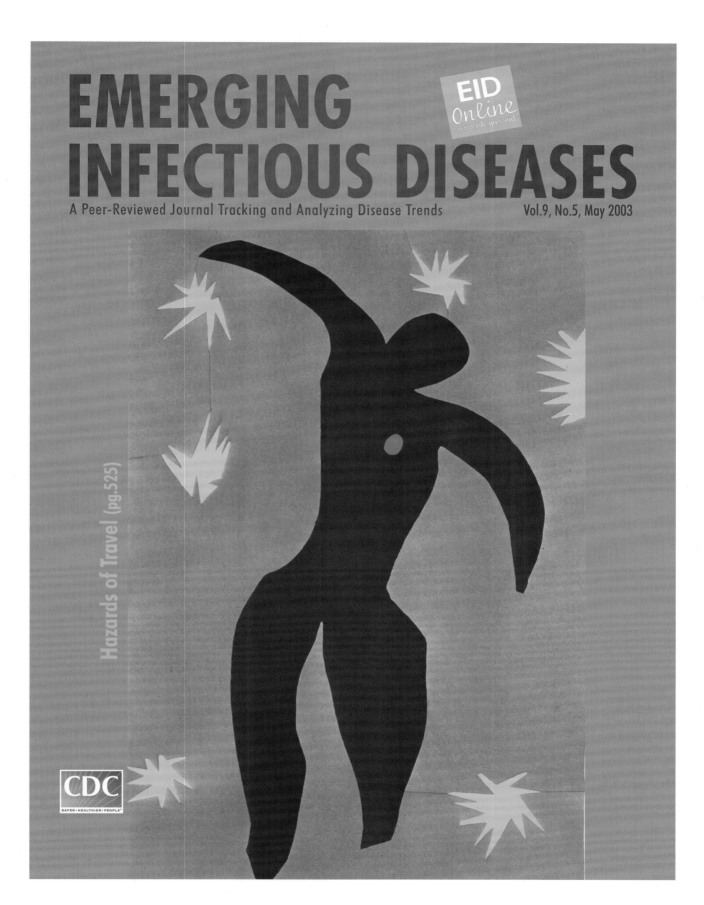

CDC
SAFER·HEALTHIER·PEOPLE™

HAZARDS OF TRAVEL

"Send me a white cane," Henri Matisse exhorted his assistants when he completed the compositions for his illustrated book *Jazz*. The artist was nearly blinded by working with intense color under the brilliant Mediterranean light of the south of France. To protect against glare, he used overstated hues and intense blacks. To overcome incapacitating illness, he invented a new medium, "drawing with scissors." Cutting shapes from prepainted paper, he formed the contour and the internal area of a shape simultaneously, eliminating as he put it, "the eternal conflict between drawing and color." These cutouts, begun as compensation for illness that confined him to a wheelchair, became another creative peak near the end of the artist's life.

Matisse started to paint while convalescing from appendicitis at age 20. He became so captivated by the joy of creative expression that within a year he abandoned his law aspirations and went to Paris to study art, in a period still reverberating with the color innovations of van Gogh, Gauguin, and Cézanne. Trained in the academic tradition by symbolist painter Gustave Moreau, Matisse used his love of the human figure and his solid footing in art history as a springboard to greatness. He became a leader of the Fauve movement, known for its radical, even violent, use of color. He broadened his artistic scope through study of Japanese prints, Persian ceramics, and Arabic designs and sought inspiration in Spain and Morocco. His long career as painter and sculptor was filled with restless experimentation, and in addition to innovative paper cutouts, his artistic efforts extended to tapestry, ceramics, stained glass, and murals. Along with Pablo Picasso, he became a pillar of 20th-century art.

In *Jazz*, Matisse's cutout forms are mingled with meditations on random topics, elaborately scrolled and interspersed throughout the composition. In this syncopated design, perhaps the visual counterpart of jazz music, which the artist defined as "rhythm and meaning," figures are chromatic and rhythmic improvisations distilled to pure form. Spare and geometric, they are filled with undulating movement and circular rhythm. Even though their range is deliberately reduced, the colors are exuberant and provocative, and the harmonious compositions are filled with almost palpable light.

In "Notes of a Painter," Matisse reflected that his goal as an artist was to uncover and record with balance and purity the "essential character" of things beneath their external appearance. *Icarus* is one of the most famous figures in *Jazz*. The cutout interprets the symbolic journey of Daedalus' son and depicts the fall of the mythological adventurer from the azure skies amidst "either stars or bursts of artillery fire" (perhaps reflecting the artist's consternation in the aftermath of World War II). The pure form of the cutout, and the color that constitutes rather than clothes the form, captures the essence of human exploration.

Icarus' stretched-out arms negotiating flight, the fiery heart cloaked in the vibrant black of its aspirations, the bright chunks of sun that proved the man's demise freeze in a moment of exhilaration. About to end, the euphoric moment turns somber. The head is tilted away from the sun's splendor toward the pedestrian view below. The gliding figure, closing its celestial dance and filled with exalted vertigo, is laden with the certainty of the fall.

Our age has transformed Icarian and heliotropic quests into space exploration. We orbit the globe, defying the sun and the forces of gravity, for we still long for the charged moment of discovery that comes from roaming the earth and beyond. Yet we have conquered neither gravity nor the mundane hazards at our destinations. Like Daedalus' crude fabrications, our wings still melt in the heat, and during travel, we fall prey to biologic hazards, exotic microbes. Be it emergent viruses, such as the cause of SARS, or common intestinal bacteria, including *Aeromonas* spp., the most insistent plague of travelers, these hazards slow the journey and limit the height of human exploration.

Bibliography

Elderfield J, dir. *Henri Matisse. Masterworks from the Museum of Modern Art*. New York, NY: The Museum of Modern Art; 1997.

Kaniamos P. The tale of Daedalus and Icarus as described in Greek mythology. Available at: http://www.skyfly.cz/zajimavo/icarus.htm. Accessed March 24, 2003.

Matisse H. *Jazz*. New York, NY: George Braziller; 1992.

EMERGING

CDC

INFECTIOUS DISEASES®

March 2009

Travel-related Emergence

Courtesy of Norton Simon Art Foundation, Pasadena, CA, USA

TANGO WITH COWS

Farm animals engaged in a sophisticated dance is how poet Vasily Kamensky represented the incongruous entanglement between Russia's rural past and sweeping modernism. In his daring book *Tango with Cows*, he abandoned syntax for a spatial arrangement of words on old wallpaper to explore visual poetry. Political oppression, industrial development, and rapid urbanization between the revolutions of 1905 and 1917 shook the foundation of society and promoted experimentation in literature, music, and art. Part of sprouting radical movements known as Russian avant-garde, Liubov Popova made her mark as a leading artist of the 20th century.

Popova was born near Moscow into an affluent family approving of her talent. She traveled widely, within Russia for the architecture and hagiography and abroad to Italy and France. She studied cubism at the Académie de la Palette under Henri Le Fauconnier and Jean Metzinger. While she admired Giotto and other masters of the Renaissance, her work moved steadily away from naturalism toward a personal style drawn from the flat linearity of Russian icons, the principles of cubism, and revolutionary ideas. "Representation of reality—without artistic deformation and transformation—cannot be the subject of painting," she wrote.

In its origins with Picasso and Braque, cubism was a formal style applied to traditional subjects to depict space and volume through multiple viewpoints and shifting planes. With time, others saw in its geometric precision the potential to capture modern life and its increasing reliance on machines. In Italy, a group called the futurists used it to express in art what Albert Einstein defined in 1905 in his theory of relativity, a new sense of time, space, and energy. "We wish to exalt aggressive movement," read the futurist manifesto, "feverish insomnia, running, the perilous leap, the cuff, and the blow." From her travels, Popova brought home these influences, which she integrated with folk and decorative elements in shaping the development of combined cubism and futurism in Russia.

She joined major art studios and worked with Vladimir Tatlin, advocate of constructivism: the exploration of geometric form in two and three dimensions, not for art's sake but as service to society. She became increasingly devoted to abstraction, and in 1916 she joined the Supremus group, organized by Kazimir Malevich: "The artist has rid himself of everything which pre-decided the objective ideal structure of life and 'art,'" he wrote. "He has freed himself from ideas, concepts and representations in order to listen only to pure sensibility."

Popova turned exclusively to dynamic geometric forms and experimented with texture, rhythm, density, and color in works she called "painterly architectonics." Unlike the painters of European cubism and futurism, who never abandoned recognizable form, she was able to develop a completely nonrepresentational idiom through layered panels of color.

The "Artist Builder," as she became known, proposed that "Form transformed is abstract and finds itself totally subject to architectonic requirements, as well as to the intentions of the artist, who attains complete freedom in total abstraction, in the distribution and construction of lines, surfaces, volumetric elements and chromatic values." Popova participated in many exhibitions and became very successful.

In 1921, she joined other artists in rejecting studio painting in favor of industrial design: textile, book, porcelain, ceramic, theater set. As a designer of women's fabrics at the First State Cotton-Printing factory, she was called upon to "unite the demands of economics, the laws of exterior design, and the mysterious taste of the peasant woman from Tula," a task she reportedly did not resent. "Not one of her artistic successes ever gave her such deep satisfaction as the sight of a peasant woman and a worker buying lengths of her material."

Popova's precipitous rise to artistic prominence was marred by infectious disease catastrophes. Her husband of 1 year, an art historian, died of typhoid fever. Infected herself, she survived, but only briefly. She died at age 35 of scarlet fever caught from her son, who died days before she did. Her untimely demise cut short a brilliant artistic career. One obituary read, "This spring, the women of Moscow . . . the cooks, the service workers—began dressing themselves up. Instead of the former petite bourgeois little flowers, there appeared on the fabrics new and unexpected strong and clear patterns."

The Traveler was painted when Popova was committed to abstraction but still maintained in her work recognizable forms. At first glance, the image appears a jumble of planes, triangles, cylinders, and semicircles arranged aggressively across the canvas to the very edge. But a closer look yields clues to an image possibly shattered and reconstructed from its fragments.

At the center of the composition, a yellow necklace draws the eye to a hidden female form. Nearby, a collar follows the curve of a cape against a cochleated armrest. The neck, head, and part of a hat are discernible. A green umbrella, firmly clutched, takes front center, its generous flaps against the passenger's legs and feet below. The seated figure delineated, the viewer can make out passing scenery: a glimpse of railing, a flag, some green. Letters are stenciled over the image forming shop signs and guideposts: "dangerous zone," "magazines," "natural gas."

Movement is achieved by overlapped planes denoting rapid succession. Shapes, tilted and angled into each other, are shaded and textured for depth and motion. Traveler and surroundings are one, gliding seamlessly in time and space.

Part and parcel of her tumultuous times, Popova recaptured in this painting not just the fragments of a broken image but also revolutionary concepts vital to science and public health. Her traveler, so directly connected with everything, carries with her everything, wherever she goes. And as she moves elegantly from place to place, she changes, as does the landscape. She is faster or slower. She picks up things from one place and deposits them in another, ambivalent about past, present, or future.

Just as the rapid influx of technology produced radical art movements, an explosion of travel around the world has irrevocably globalized everything, dragging the rural cow into the metropolitan area to tango. The close meeting of different worlds, back and forth, from country to country and countryside to city, is making the old from the old environment ripe for emergence of the new in a new environment.

Bibliography

Bowlt J, Drutt M, eds. *Amazons of the Avant-Garde*. New York, NY: Guggenheim Museum; 1999.

Dabrowski M. *Liubov Popova*. New York, NY: Museum of Modern Art; 1991.

Elderfield J, ed. *Modern Painting and Sculpture*. New York, NY: Museum of Modern Art; 2004.

Fer B, Batchelor D, Wood P. *Realism, Rationalism, Surrealism: Art between the Wars*. New Haven, CT: Yale University Press in association with the Open University; 1994.

J. Paul Getty Museum. Tango with cows: book art of the Russian avant-guarde, 1910–1917. Available at: http://www.getty.edu/art/exhibitions/tango_with_cows/curators_essay.html. Accessed January 22, 2009.

EMERGING
INFECTIOUS DISEASES

EID Online www.cdc.gov/eid

A Peer-Reviewed Journal Tracking and Analyzing Disease Trends   Vol.11, No.1, January 2005

Foodborne Disease

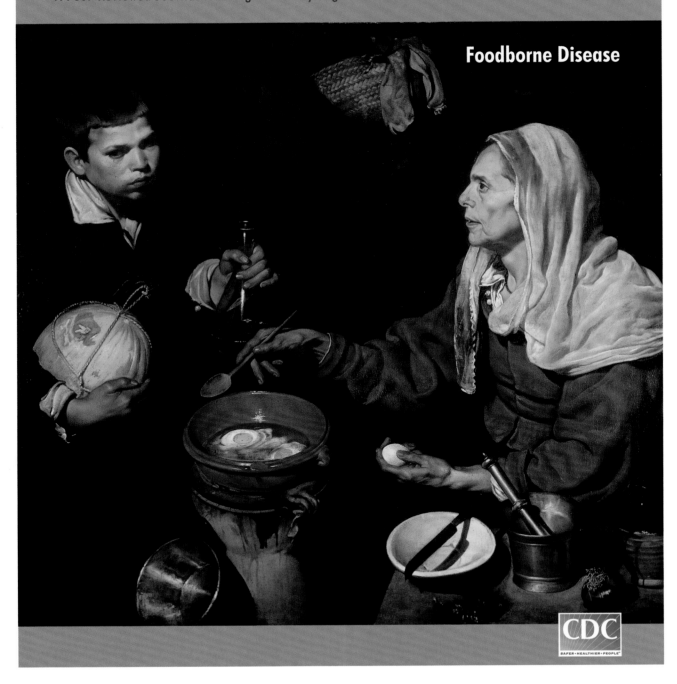

CDC
SAFER • HEALTHIER • PEOPLE

GENRE PAINTING AND THE WORLD'S KITCHEN

"Tell me what you eat, I will tell you who you are," boasted famed gastronome Jean Anthelme Brillat-Savarin (1755–1826). A man of many interests, among them archaeology, astronomy, and chemistry, Savarin wrote treatises on economics and history, but his fascination with food was what most informed and entertained readers and followers in his native France and around the world. In nature and on the table, quite apart from its direct link to human survival, food has been an object of intrigue featured prominently in art throughout history. From ancient times and particularly during the development of genre painting in the Middle Ages and later, food—its appearance, abundance, or decay—has been a popular subject.

In 17th-century Spain, genre painting reached new heights with the work of Diego Velázquez. In a style reminiscent of Caravaggio, Velázquez created and popularized the kitchen or tavern scene (*bodegón*), which showed peasants eating or preparing meals and the objects they used to assemble and serve them. These objects, prominently displayed in realistic terms including their imperfections, assumed a life of their own, introducing a new naturalism in Spanish painting, which had been dominated by the ideal beauty of classical and academic themes.

Velázquez grew up in the cosmopolitan climate of Seville, southern Spain, along the banks of the Guadalquivir, an area also home to Cervantes, Lope de Vega, and other luminaries of the Spanish Golden Age. Like the great literature of that era, his art concerned itself with the life, culture, and traditions of the people. He apprenticed with influential biographer, theoretician, and artist Francisco Pacheco, who later wrote about his student: "After five years of education and training, I married him to my daughter, moved by his virtue, integrity, and good parts and by the expectations of his disposition and great talent."

Soon a member of the Seville painters' guild, Velázquez moved from *bodegón* to portraits and was summoned to the court, where he received his first commission to paint King Philip IV, a discerning patron of the arts. He was appointed court painter, a position of great privilege, which gave him access to royal collections, including paintings by the Venetian Renaissance master Titian, who greatly influenced the development of his style. The artist led a quiet life, interrupted only by his travels to Italy, sponsored by the king. During his first journey, he traveled with Flemish Baroque master Peter Paul Rubens, who was also influential in his artistic career.

"To go to Madrid to see the Velázquez" was Monet's wish near the end of his life. This wish, expressed in a letter to a friend, reflects the mystique associated with Velázquez's work and the breadth of its influence on all modern art schools, even if limited to 100 or so surviving works. His painting showed exceptional mastery of space and light and exuded naturalness and restraint, both in its objectivity and choice of colors, often browns and ochers. Velázquez was gifted with exacting technique and preferred to paint from life. In spite of his meticulous depiction of reality, he seemed more interested in the tensions between reality and appearance than in reality itself.

Velásquez painted *An Old Woman Cooking Eggs* when he was 19 years old. In this kitchen scene, the common utensils used in preparing food (mortar and pestle, pots, ladles, bowl, jugs) have at least as important a place as the preparers themselves.

Provocatively in the foreground and along the edges of the painting, these objects seem to contain in their clay, wood, glass, brass, copper, pewter, or other essence the light that defines them against the dark background. The eggshell, the straw of the basket, the skin of the melon and onion, the texture of linen and string, showcase the artist's virtuoso performance in capturing their likeness.

The food preparers, transfixed by some unknown concern, seem removed and distant from the food and from each other. They go through the motions of cooking, but their minds are elsewhere. The boy, cradling a trussed melon, leans forward with a glass cruet containing oil, wine, or some other liquid. The old woman tending the food is staring intently ahead, otherwise preoccupied. On a ceramic heating plate, the pan is tipped forward to show the eggs in various stages of congealing. The curved shadow of the knife over the bowl, the moist surface of the pan above the egg whites, the gleaming copper pot against the shadows of the room confirm the artist's interest in the integrity and dignity of these objects and the people who use them, even if he does not indulge us with their concerns underneath the surface.

These concerns, apart from the underlying threat of decay through the relentless passage of time, a common theme in still-life painting, would be many, even if they were only limited to food. The 17th-century Spanish diet was known for its parsimony. A main concern in the common kitchen was the long-term availability of food. The safety of food, a more modern concern, was probably not on the mind of Velásquez's food preparers. Unlike our contemporary equivalents, they would have known little about the dangers surrounding food. Nor would they have understood Savarin, whose sensitive 18th-century palate might have recoiled at the sight of eggs poaching slowly in oil on a clay stove.

An ancient staple, eggs have run the gamut from plentiful protein to gourmet delicacy. Yet basic food and epicurean aspirations converge at one point: safety. With high levels of *Salmonella enterica* serovar Enteriditis in shell eggs, adequate cooking and proper temperature of the eggs overrule tradition, challenging the consistency of the sauce and the moment of delivery to the table. In our times, safety issues concerning not only eggs but all foods beg a different interpretation of another well-known Savarin aphorism, "The destiny of a nation depends on the manner in which it feeds itself."

Bibliography

Brillat-Savarin JA. *Physiologie du Gout*. Paris, France: Feydeau; 1826.

Portús J. *Velásquez*. Barcelona, Spain: Aldeasa; 2000.

Schroeder CM, Naugle AL, Schlosser WD, et al. Estimate of illnesses from *Salmonella* Enteriditis in eggs, United States, 2000. *Emerg Infect Dis.* 2004;12:116–118.

Web Gallery of Art. Baroque painting: the Golden Age. Available at: http://www.wga.hu/tours/spain/p_17.html. Accessed April 24, 2013.

EMERGING
INFECTIOUS DISEASES®

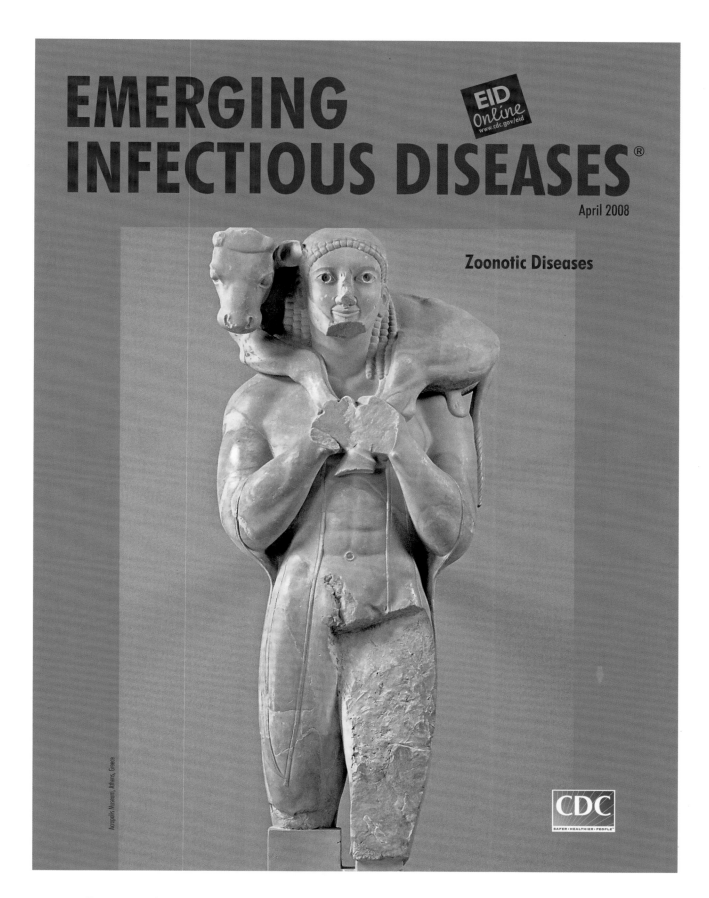

EID Online www.cdc.gov/eid

April 2008

Zoonotic Diseases

Acropolis Museum, Athens, Greece

CDC
SAFER · HEALTHIER · PEOPLE™

IN DREAMS BEGIN RESPONSIBILITIES[1]

"I woke with this marble head in my hands; / It exhausts my elbows and I don't know where to put it down. / It was falling into the dream as I was coming out of the dream / So our life became one and it will be very difficult for it to separate again," wrote George Seferis about his relationship with art from antiquity. Traversing the edges of time has long been the domain of artists and poets, who view history as a continuous process not to be fragmented and labeled "ancient" as if somehow interrupted or expired.

"The art of [marble] sculpture is much older than that of painting or bronze statuary," wrote Pliny the Elder. Early sculptors worked on marble with point chisels, punches, and stone abrasives. Repeated vertical blows shattered crystals deep into the stone, altering the outer gloss. Because statues were painted, the opaque surface benefited pigment application. On the Acropolis, the first marble statues appeared more 2,000 years ago. They were votives, mostly maidens called *kores* but also young men, *kouri*. Some were inscribed with the names of artists; others, with dedications. They represented the donor or a deity, a renowned athlete, or the deceased if intended for a gravesite. They dominated art of the archaic period. Thousands have been excavated from various sites.

Neither gods nor mortals, *kores* and *kouri* embodied physical perfection accessible to both. They were free-standing, the earliest such examples of large stone images of the human form in the history of art. Their arms were separated from the torso, the legs from each other. Tense and filled with life, they had various faces and expressions, their individuality foreshadowing portraiture. Their large eyes stared directly ahead, and they were injected with emotion, the stylized "archaic smile," signifying not happiness but emerging humanity. They wore flowing garments, carefully delineated, and appeared refreshed and carefree, as if suddenly become aware of themselves.

The best known of these figures, *Moschophoros* (calf-bearer), represented the donor, a nobleman named Romvos as inscribed on the base. The figure, found in fragments on the grounds of the Acropolis near the sanctuary of the Temple of Athena, has none of the masklike quality of earlier *kouri*. Though he has their usual left-foot-forward stance and stylized tufted hair, *Moschophoros* is not a youth but a mature man with a beard. His fitted cloak was likely painted in vivid colors as were the lips and hair. "The hollow eyes . . . once held inlays of semi-precious stones (mother-of-pearl, gray agate, or lapis lazuli) that would have given the face a strikingly realistic appearance."

Romvos is carrying an animal for sacrifice on the altar of Goddess Athena, a formidable fixture of the Hellenic pantheon known for its temperamental deities and countless demigods and their descendents. Their origins and relationships with humans were fodder for myths and art through sculpture and elaborate iconography. Gods gave gifts and favors. Humans offered votives as thanks, atonement, entreaty, or worship.

---

1 William Butler Yeats, *Responsibilities.*

Sacrifice (from sacrificium [sacred] + facere [make] = to make sacred) was a central part of religious practice during festivals and feast days. The ritual was performed in well-defined space within a temple sanctuary. Some feasts were Pan-Hellenic and included processions and athletic competitions. "There are sanctuaries of Hermes Kriophoros," wrote Pausanias, describing the city of Tanagra. "Hermes averted a pestilence from the city by carrying a ram round the walls; to commemorate this Calamis made an image of Hermes carrying a ram upon his shoulders. Whichever of the youths is judged to be the most handsome goes round the walls at the feast carrying a lamb on his shoulders."

Homer mentions sacrifice "of bulls, of goats" in *The Iliad* and of "sleek black bulls to Poseidon, god of the seablue mane who shakes the earth," in *The Odyssey*. The most common offering was the sheep, goat, or pig, but the ox and bull were also used, depending on the occasion. Animals were selected for their physical perfection, their horns gilded and adorned with ribbons and garlands. As the animal walked toward the altar, barley was thrown in its path to entice it and water sprinkled on its head, causing it to nod as in agreement with the proceedings. The crowd was silent, then sorrowful, acknowledging the sacrifice. The ritual turned into a feast, "while the people tasted the innards, burned the thighbones for the god" (*The Odyssey*, Book III).

The contradictions inherent in religious sacrifice did not elude ritual participants, who ate little meat outside these religious feasts. The rituals may have expressed their uneasiness at killing animals for food and to appease the gods. Their ambivalence continued during the classical period, when even large domestic animals sustainable only in small numbers were used. "Our ancestors handed down to us the most powerful and prosperous community . . . by performing the prescribed sacrifices," wrote Athens orator Lysias, defending the practice. "It is therefore proper for us to offer the same . . . if only for the sake of the success which has resulted from those rites."

Moschophoros stuns for its ability to bring to life eons after its creation a moment of connection. The human face, wearing a smile, the single most appealing adornment then and now, is framed by the surrendered animal. The marble seems to melt in the calf's unparalleled fragility and tenderness. Locked in a secure embrace, human and animal take a step together, an ear touching, a tail relaxed.

"My pawing over the ancients and semi-ancients," wrote Ezra Pound, "has been one long struggle to find out what has been done, once for all, better than it can ever be done again, and to find out what remains for us to do." *Moschophoros* captured the primeval ease between man and calf. What remains to do? For us the challenge is to get beyond the sacrifice. Whether to appease the gods or stop bovine spongiform encephalopathy, charred remains of cattle and other animals betray limited success in our symbiotic relationship. Increased animal translocation and ecologic transformation add to the intrigue, along with microbial changes now seen at the molecular level.

Moschophoros is not ancient. The statue exists in the present. It can be touched, viewed, and examined for universal meaning. Resilient and unchanged, it defies death. And like other marvels from antiquity, it takes the initiative in speaking to us. "The statues are not the ruins," wrote Seferis, "—we are the ruins."

Bibliography

Dontas G. *The Acropolis and Its Museum*. Douma A, trans. Athens, Greece: Clio Editions; 1979.

Eliot TS, ed. *Literary Essays of Ezra Pound*. New York, NY: New Directions; 1968.

Fiero GK. *The Humanistic Tradition, Books 1–6*. New York, NY: McGraw-Hill Humanities/ Social Studies/Languages; 2001.

Keeley E. George Seferis, the art of poetry no. 13. *The Paris Review*. Available at: http://www. theparisreview.com/viewinterview.php/prmMID/4112. Accessed February 20, 2008.

Martin TR. An overview of classical Greek history from Mycenae to Alexander. Available at: http://www.perseus.tufts.edu/hopper/text?doc=Perseus%3Atext%3A1999.04.0009&redi rect=true. Accessed February 20, 2007.

Pausanias. *Description of Greece*. Jones WHS, trans. Cambridge, MA: Harvard University Press and London, England: William Heinemann; 1918.

Pliny the Elder. *Natural History*. Healey JF, trans. London, England: Penguin Classics; 1991.

Seferis G. Mythistorima. In: Keeley E, Sherrard P, eds. *Collected Poems of George Seferis*. Princeton, NJ: Princeton University Press; 1995.

Vol 10, No 12, December 2004

EMERGING INFECTIOUS DISEASES

A Peer-Reviewed Journal Tracking and Analyzing Disease Trends   Vol.10, No.12, December 2004

EID Online
www.cdc.gov/eid

Zoonotic Diseases

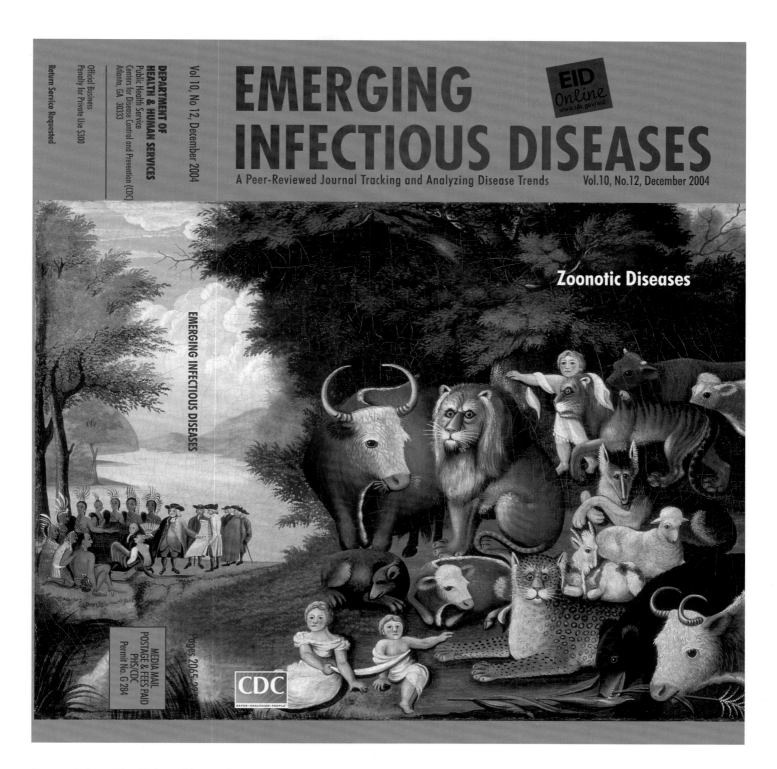

DEPARTMENT OF
HEALTH & HUMAN SERVICES
Public Health Service
Centers for Disease Control and Prevention (CDC)
Atlanta, GA 30333

Official Business
Penalty for Private Use $300

Return Service Requested

EMERGING INFECTIOUS DISEASES

MEDIA MAIL
POSTAGE & FEES PAID
PHS/CDC
Permit No. G 284

Pages 2065–

CDC
SAFER·HEALTHIER·PEOPLE™

"ONE MEDICINE" FOR ANIMAL AND HUMAN HEALTH

"The wolf also shall dwell with the lamb, and the leopard shall lie down with the kid, the calf, and the young lion, and the fatling together, and a little child shall lead them." These biblical lines (Isaiah 11:6–9) provided Edward Hicks the allegorical framework in which to approach a theme of special fascination to him: the peaceable kingdom, an idyllic world in which all creatures live in harmony. He painted more than 100 versions of this theme, 62 of which have survived.

A native of Bucks County, Pennsylvania, Hicks was orphaned in infancy and raised by a Quaker family. At 13 years of age, he was apprenticed to a carriage maker and learned to decorate coaches. He showed natural talent for decorative painting and, even without academic training, became very successful. "I am now employing four hands, besides myself, in coach, sign and ornamental painting, and still more in repairing and finishing carriages," he wrote reflecting on his experiences, "and I think I should find no difficulty in doubling my business."

As a young man, Hicks set out to explore the wild side of life but soon returned to the Quakers and became a popular itinerant preacher. This Religious Society of Friends espoused the principles of equality and nonviolence but frowned upon artistic ventures as too worldly. Hicks abandoned his ornamental painting business to become a farmer only to relent, reluctantly, in middle age and move from commercial decoration to easel painting. Inspiration came mostly from his religious faith and missionary work among Native American tribes.

Born into a new nation, just 4 years after the Declaration of Independence, Hicks became part of an 18th- and 19th-century American tradition that produced provincial or folk art (portraits, landscapes, religious, historical themes) characterized by a naïve style. This style, the hallmark of self-taught artists who arrived at their art through a journey of discovery and realization of innate talent, often flourished in rural areas and small towns. Outside traditional rules of perspective and proportion, naïve style relied on intuitive organization and structure, and was imaginative, creative, and direct.

Even though in his day he gained notoriety as an impassioned preacher, Hicks is now remembered for his art. His paintings, a continuation of his religious beliefs, explored ethical and spiritual dilemmas and commemorated historical events. Human figures, animals, and landscapes were created to embody Quaker ideals. Color, size, proportion, placement, and other elements were used as symbols to compose a moral message, which was often inscribed on the frame.

In a world marred by strife—between nations, between animals and humans, between animals themselves—Hicks tapped into the universal wish for harmony and peace. Well ahead of his time, he invited to his kingdoms not only leading human figures and innocent children but also a consortium of animals whose presence he found indispensable. Domesticated animals, part of his life as a farmer, appeared in realistic detail, but wild beasts were more idealized and decorative.

In *The Peaceable Kingdom*, Hicks once more assembled the world's creatures for an idyllic group portrait. Against a lighted backdrop of trees and river banks, animals and children gathered in the foreground. In mid-panel, leading Quaker

William Penn concluded a peace treaty with the Lenni Lenape tribe. The colors were solid, the light well focused, and the curves of animal frames and horns gracefully outlined. Yet Hicks was not denying tensions in the universe.

The animals, whose anthropomorphic features betrayed human emotions, seemed puzzled and apprehensive. Even as the bull offered the lion hay, the king of beasts seemed stiff and uneasy. Even as the lamb cuddled up, the wolf wore a noncommittal glare. The world's creatures may have been tamed, but peace in the scene seems precarious.

The connectivity that Hicks sensed between humans, animals, and the universe was greater than the artist could have imagined. The intensity in the animals' eyes was not the only troubling element in the picture. In the dander and under their breath, in the soil and in the water, on the leaves and the clothing of the dignitaries, lay creatures unknown to Hicks: microorganisms, insidiously moving from animals to humans, eating, multiplying, sharing, spreading, connecting. Even if Hicks could have arranged a perfectly peaceable kingdom, strife would have continued beneath the surface through the transmission of disease.

Not long after Hicks's death in 1849, German pathologist Rudolf Virchow (1821–1902) coined the term *zoonosis*, verifying the essential link between animal and human health. This link, further complicated by the emerging nature of disease and the ethical, ecologic, social, and economic values placed on the relation between humans and their pets, livestock, or fellow inhabitants of nature, has not been uniformly acknowledged or exploited—even in the face of AIDS, Ebola, West Nile virus, avian influenza, bovine spongiform encephalopathy, and SARS.

In the 1980s, American epidemiologist Calvin Schwabe proposed a unified human and veterinary approach against zoonotic diseases. This approach, "one medicine," upholds Virchow's principles and affirms Hicks's wish for the control of subversive elements, whether they interfere with harmonious animal and human interaction or disrupt animal and human health.

Bibliography
Bishop R, Coblentz P. *Folk Painters of America*. New York, NY: E.P. Dutton; 1979.
Saunders LZ. Virchow's contributions to veterinary medicine. *Vet Pathol*. 2000;37:199–207.
Schwabe C. *Veterinary Medicine and Human Health*. 3rd ed. Baltimore, MD: Williams and Wilkins; 1984.

EMERGING
INFECTIOUS DISEASES®

Emerging Viruses

April 2013

CDC
SAFER·HEALTHIER·PEOPLE™

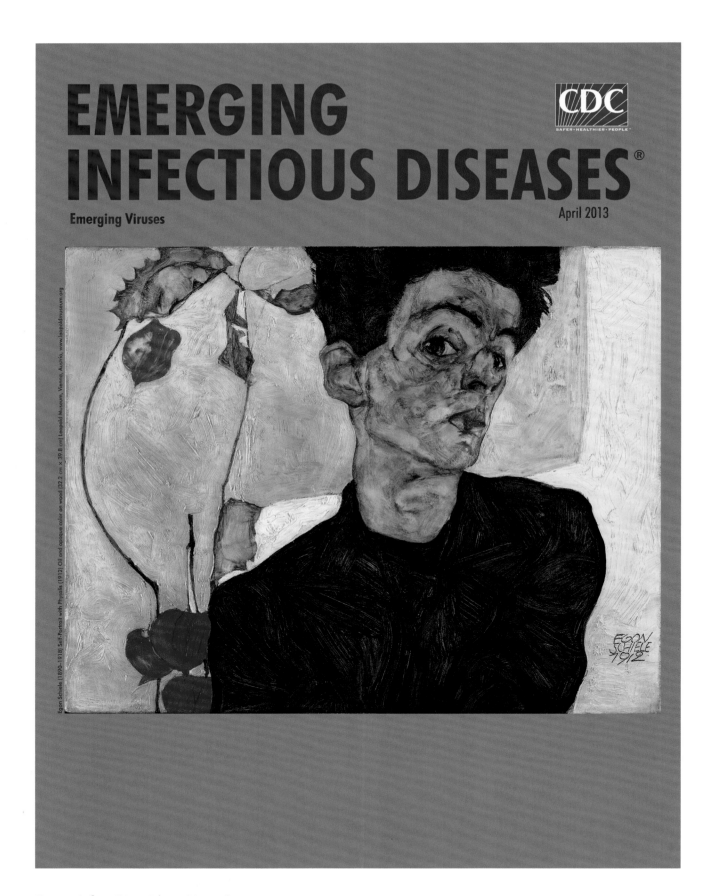

Egon Schiele (1890–1918) Self-Portrait with Physalis (1912) Oil and opaque color on wood (32.2 cm x 39.8 cm) Leopold Museum, Vienna, Austria, www.leopoldmuseum.org

PALE HORSE, PALE RIDER DONE TAKEN MY LOVER AWAY[2]

"It simply divided my life, cut across it like that. So that everything before that was just getting ready, and after that I was in some strange way altered, really," said Katherine Anne Porter about her nearly fatal encounter with the Spanish flu. "It took me a long time to go out and live in the world again." Years later, in a thinly disguised autobiographical novel, she laid out not just her own traumatic run-in with death, the pale rider, but also a rare literary account of the 1918 flu pandemic in the United States and the unprecedented human loss.

For her recollection of the pandemic, Porter had to rely on fragments of memory before her illness and after her recovery. These fragments involved the landlady; her beloved fiancé, Adam; and fatal flu in Denver, Colorado, during World War I, which killed many young men needed for battle. "I tell you, they must come for her *now* or I'll put her on the sidewalk." "They can't get an ambulance, and there aren't any beds. And we can't find a doctor or nurse. They're all busy." "It's as bad as anything can be . . . all the theaters and nearly all the shops and restaurants are closed, and the streets have been full of funerals all day and ambulances all night." "Two cherry flavored pills," "orange juice and ice cream," "coffee in a thermos bottle." "The men are dying like flies out there. . . . This funny new disease. Simply knocks you into a cocked hat."

Porter wakes up from her illness to find that Adam, "tall and heavily muscled in the shoulders, narrow in the waist and flanks," handsome Adam with "his eyes pale tan with orange flecks in them, and his hair the color of a haystack when you turn the weathered top back to the clear straw beneath," Adam, who had "never had a pain in his life that he [could] remember," had died.

Porter, the consummate storyteller, used words to express the devastating effects of illness on her life. Across the world, in Austria, Egon Schiele, whose self-portrait graces this section's cover, in similar circumstances, found no comfort in words, despite his own poetic nature. When his wife was dying of the flu, he was unable to articulate his feelings. In a letter to his mother, he coolly speculated that Edith would probably not survive. But he used art to express his devastation. He made several sketches of his wife during the last 2 days of her life. In these sketches, the lines were fluid and sensitive, the colors subdued, the format understated. All these features, a departure from his usual provocative style, reflected the emotional stability found in his life with Edith. His last work was a portrait of his wife, who died the following day. She was 6 months pregnant. He died 3 days later.

Even before his fatal encounter with the flu, Schiele was acquainted with adversity. His early years were marred by a troubled relationship with his mother, poor academic performance, and the loss of his father, a provincial railroad station-master, to tertiary syphilis, when Egon was 14 years old. "I don't know whether

---

2 Negro spiritual, in Katherine Anne Porter's *Pale Horse, Pale Rider*. See also "Go Down Death: A Funeral Sermon" in *God's Trombones: Seven Negro Sermons in Verse* at http://docsouth.unc.edu/southlit/johnson/johnson.html

there is anyone else at all who remembers my noble father with such sadness." The elder Schiele had kept his condition from his 17-year-old bride, Egon's mother. Her first three babies were stillborn. The fourth child died at age 10 of meningitis, a complication of late-onset congenital syphilis. Egon was the first boy to survive. "I shall be the fruit which after its decay will leave behind eternal life; therefore how great must be your joy—to have borne me?" Egon wrote to his mother. His penchant for grandiosity and certain physical features in his early self-portraits led some to wonder whether he might have also been infected.

Schiele lived his life at an accelerated pace. He started to draw as a child and was enrolled in the Vienna Academy of Fine Arts at age 16. He became a protégé of Gustav Klimt, a strong early influence. Once when asked whether young Schiele's drawings showed talent, Klimt responded, "Much too much." The gifted but troublesome student would soon go off on his own and form the New Artists group. Later, when Klimt was struck down by the flu, Schiele made several portraits of him on his deathbed.

Schiele went on to serve in the military; to have high-profile love affairs; get arrested and be thrown in jail; and before his own untimely death, make a proper and by all accounts promising marriage. All along, he grew as an artist and achieved an expressionist style focused on feelings and their interpretation. He was drawn to the unconventional and controversial, and his hundreds of self-portraits were penetrating and disquieting. His exaggerated lines, unrealistic shapes, and intense colors invoked human situations with a candor that many found disturbing. During his brief career he created more than 3,000 works on paper, some 300 paintings. Despite the edginess, his artistic reputation grew, he was offered commissions, and his work sold well.

In interpreting any self-portrait, it is tempting to draw clues from the artist's life. During his short career, Schiele was alienated and vulnerable and in the midst of World War I and pandemic flu. *Self-Portrait with Physalis*, probably his best-known self-portrait, shows him at the peak of his creativity in 1912, his most productive year, when his expressionist style had matured. Clues for interpreting a self-portrait can also be drawn from facial expressions, gestures, and props within the painting—what the artist allows us to see. In this self-portrait, the arms and body are severely cropped, only the cocked head and shoulders are shown. The one-eyed stare challenges the viewer. So do the pursed lips. This is a laconic composition, though a theatrical one, what with its intensely colored lampion fruit and dreamy sentimentality. Despite the scattered character clues, there is one thing we will never know from Schiele's *Self-Portrait with Physalis*, and that is what would have happened if he had not died at age 28 of pandemic flu.

When the pandemic ended, which took away even her "decrepit hound and silver kitten," there was, Porter wrote, a "dazed silence." The "Great Pandemic" claimed more lives in a short time than any other disease in history, yet because it was intertwined with the "Great War," the horror of it in human terms may not have been adequately chronicled. Some have called it the "forgotten pandemic"—but not those who work in public health.

Many strides have been made in flu prevention and control since 1918: better understanding of the virus, its distribution in nature, its presence in animals and birds, some of its virulence factors, how it mutates, how it is distributed in tissues, how it is transmitted. We now have prevention programs, vaccines, and antiviral drugs. But many still die, and the threat of another pandemic lurks.

Dramatic tension captured in literature and art prevents us from forgetting the dead and the grave pandemics of history. Schiele did his part by immortalizing the faces of his beloved persons—very much like Porter who, in her version of the spiritual "Pale Horse, Pale Rider," contends that death takes away the singer's lover, mother, siblings, and eventually over the course of several verses the entire family, "But not the singer, not yet," "Death always leaves one singer to mourn." That's to ensure remembrance, which applies as well in public health, where to prevent the next pandemic, it pays to remember and study the past ones.

Bibliography

Chandra S. Deaths associated with influenza pandemic of 1918–19, Japan. *Emerg Infect Dis.* 2013;19:616–622.

Comini A. *Egon Schiele: Portraits*. Berkeley, CA: University of California Press; 1974.

Fuller TL, Gilbert M, Martin V, et al. Predicting hotspots for influenza reassortment. *Emerg Infect Dis.* 2013;19:581–588.

Kallir J. *Egon Schiele: Life and Work*. New York, NY: Harry N Abrams; 2003.

Knafo D. *Egon Schiele: A Self in Creation: A Psychoanalytic Study of the Artist's Self-Portraits*. Madison, NJ: Fairleigh Dickinson University Press; 1993.

Kuster SP, Coleman BL, Raboud J, et al. Risk factors for influenza infection among health care workers during 2009 pandemic, Toronto, Ontario, Canada. *Emerg Infect Dis.* 2013; 19:606–615.

Lekana-Douki SE, Mouinga-Ondémé A, Nkoghe D, et al. Early introduction and delayed dissemination of pandemic influenza, Gabon. *Emerg Infect Dis.* 2013;19:644–647.

Lucie-Smith E. *Lives of the Great 20th-Century Artists*. London, England: Thames and Hudson; 1999.

Porter KA. *Pale Horse, Pale Rider: Three Short Novels*. New York, NY: Harcourt, Brace; 1939.

Taubenberger JK, Reid AH, Lourens RM, et al. Characterization of the 1918 influenza virus polymerase genes. *Nature*. 2005;437:889–893.

EMERGING
INFECTIOUS DISEASES®

March 2007

Extensively Drug-resistant TB

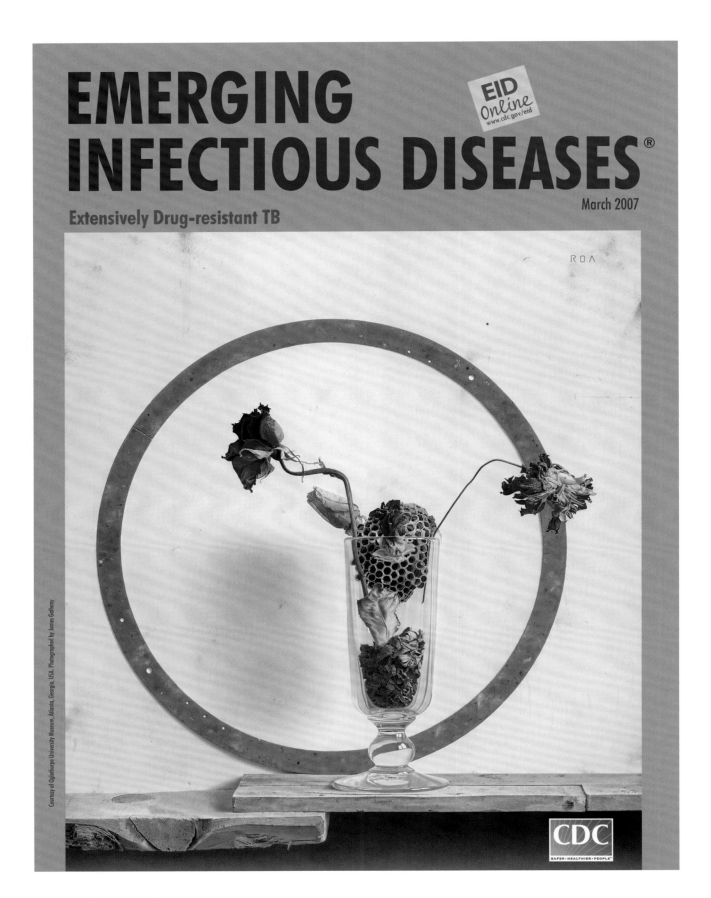

Courtesy of Oglethorpe University Museum, Atlanta, Georgia, USA. Photographed by James Gathany

THE WAY FORWARD IS THE WAY BACK[3]

"The viewer should see the object as I saw it, but with a lot of room for his own interpretation. . . . The painting is like a very clear mirror which is barely visible but unmistakably there," reflects Spanish painter Antonio López García (b. 1936). "I am nostalgic for an art of our times in which a greater number of people can participate." Part of a contemporary movement rooted in the traditions of 17th-century Spanish realism, López García, Claudio Bravo, Bern Tanodrroens, Francisco Roa, and many others have drawn inspiration from the meticulous work of Francisco de Zurbarán, Jusepe de Ribera, and Diego Velásquez to create their own naturalist style.

Rejecting abstraction, these artists create paintings from a broad range of subjects, choosing, much like their predecessors, a few or even one subject, which they lavish with extreme seriousness and attention, focusing on the "credible detail, that small touch of the familiar," that has long been part of the repertory of Spanish painters. The characteristic high technical quality is not an end in itself, and the work reaches far beyond mere representation of nature.

In the United States, revival of traditional painting skills in the latter part of the 20th century is credited to professor Richard Lack, who in his essay "On the Training of Painters" (1969) envisioned atelier training in the contemporary art scene. "Indeed if Western Civilization wishes to retain the art of painting as a living part of its culture, this may be our last hope." He founded the pioneering Atelier Lack in Minneapolis, "a small island of traditional art training surrounded by a sea of hostile opinion." Rigorous technique, which had fallen by the wayside in modern times, addressed quality of drawing, color plausibility, truthfulness of light and shadow, highly developed skills of execution, and overall faithful depiction of nature.

The atelier attracted students from all over the world and became the model for similar schools, among them The New York Academy of Art and the Charles H. Cecil Studios in Florence, Italy. The New York Academy of Art won the support of Andy Warhol: "The course of art history," he said, "would be changed if one thousand students could be taught Old Master drawing and painting techniques."

In 1982, Lack coined the term "Classical Realism" because as he put it, "Any 20th-century painting that suggests a recognizable object, however crudely or childishly rendered, qualifies as 'realistic.' Obviously, the simple word 'realism,' when applied to painting . . . is no longer meaningful." But contemporary American realists are a disparate group, loosely characterized by a realistic approach to representation, which has persisted widely in the post-abstraction era.

A painter in the tradition of Spanish realism, Francisco Roa was born in Guadalajara, Spain, and moved to Madrid at age 18 to study at the Universidad Complutense and the Academia Peña. He has received considerable recognition at home, exhibiting in Madrid, Barcelona, and Granada. In 1993, he took his works to Lisbon and Miami, and a year later, to New York and Atlanta.

Extremely careful with detail, Roa, like many of his contemporaries, conveys an individual perception of reality, positioning everyday objects deliberately, proposing

---

3 Herakleitos of Ephesus, c. 2,500 years ago.

his own space and time. *Sands Flowers*, first exhibited in the United States in 1994, is a characteristic still life.

Against a vacant background vaguely reminiscent of sand, the artist composes a geometric ensemble to anchor his main object of interest, a glass vessel filled with natural elements past their prime. The board base, stacked on the left, breaks up the horizontal field. The metal circle, weathered and discolored, is slightly of center, the backdrop deliberately smudged. Inside the glass lie red petals, crinkled and lifeless, the detritus of beauty. Crammed in near the top is a hornet's nest, and out of each side, dried blooms jut pathetically, their stems distorted and petals curled.

"All forms of beauty, like all possible phenomena," wrote Charles Baudelaire in his *On the Heroism of Modern Life*, "contain an element of the eternal and an element of the transitory—of the absolute and the particular." In a perfect balance of feeling and form, Roa's poignant scene meets Baudelaire's requirement. For nothing expresses the ephemeral better than flowers. Roses or sand verbenas, they perish all too soon, a metaphor for human transience and fragility.

The eternal and the absolute are elements artists have sought in the formalities of realism and the fragments of abstraction, on the same pathway, one step forward, two steps back; and scientists likewise, for rarely does excellent science or art occur without reference to past knowledge and principle.

In *Sands Flowers*, Roa probes the precariousness of existence, space and time, life and death. His realistic representation of natural objects in decline provokes speculation—not only on the passage of time and inevitability of death, but for us, also on disease, which unduly hastens the process. In an unending circle, old scourges become new, among them tuberculosis, a hornet's nest of multiple drug resistance, and now extensive resistance to second-line drugs, raising the specter of potentially untreatable disease. Roa sought essence in the staying power of exacting detail. In science, too, on the same pathway, sometimes solutions lie simply in the core values: treatment standards, effective precautions, improved technology, better medicines, vaccines, and diagnostic tests.

Bibliography

Brenson M, Serraller FC, Sullivan EJ. *Antonio López García*. New York, NY: Rizzoli; 1990.

Brown J. *The Golden Age of Spanish Painting*. New Haven, CT: Yale University Press; 1991.

Gjertson S. Richard F. *Lack: An American Master*. Minneapolis, MN: American Society of Classical Realism; 2001.

Hedberg G. A new direction in art education. In: *Slow Painting: A Deliberate Renaissance*. Atlanta, GA: Oglethorpe University Museum of Art; 2006.

Nick L, Villalba G. *Four from Madrid: Contemporary Spanish Realism*. Atlanta, GA: Oglethorpe University Museum of Art; 1994.

Shah NS, Wright A, Bai GH, et al. Worldwide emergence of extensively drug-resistant tuberculosis. *Emerg Infect Dis*. 2007;13:380–387.

Poverty and Conflict

"I think of my work as an inhabited landscape, never static or empty. . . . The wind ruffles; ants crawl; a rabbit burrows," says Jaune Quick-to-See Smith (b. 1940), a painter of Salish, French-Cree, and Shoshone heritage. Feeling and astute observation characterize her representational, abstract, and symbolic landscapes. A prolific artist, inspired by the formal innovations of Pablo Picasso, Paul Klee, and others, she uses paint, collage, and other media to compose unique forms on tactile surfaces that explore the continuum of life, the connection between living beings and the land, and the fundamental relationship between all things. As artist, curator, and lecturer, she has promoted understanding and reverence of nature, articulated Native aesthetic tradition in a modern art context, and made her mark on the contemporary American art scene.

Native American cultures did not refer to art as a separate discipline before the mid-19th century. Cultural materials with aesthetic value (totem poles, pottery, beadwork) were integrated into everyday life and traditional practices. Artists painted geometric patterns or symbolic representations of figures on readily available media (sand, hides, clay); wood, bone, and stone were carved for a three-dimensional effect. The iconography and function of the work varied widely with region and tribe, but all objects were imbued with spirituality and were meant to serve the community.

Serving the community, so important in Native culture, presupposes a well-functioning and productive group. Yet the community can be disrupted by poverty and disease. Emerging infections cause social inequity and are caused by it. As illness and premature death increase, health care systems struggle to keep up with the costs, and services erode even further. Deaths among the poor, especially among women, children, and the elderly, are disproportionately high since these groups' access to medical attention and prevention measures, such as vaccination, is inadequate. Remedios Varo's *La Llamada* (*The Call*) draws attention to the plight of those overlooked by the health care communities. Bartolomé Esteban Murillo's *The Young Beggar* completes the discussion with its emphasis on the plight of children overlooked and abandoned by societies.

The breakdown of public health measures, with its consequent unsanitary conditions, poor hygiene, lack of potable water, and suspended immunizations and disease control, fuels the emergence of infections around the world. In the United

States, it has at times caused the reemergence of measles, a vaccine-preventable childhood disease; inadequate vaccine supplies for other preventable diseases; increases in health care–related infections from poor infection-control practices; lower immunization rates; and decreased availability of experts in vector control for such diseases as West Nile encephalitis. Jacob Lawrence's *Marionettes* provides the backdrop for examining the hopelessness and despair among those who are caught in the unending cycle of poverty and disease.

Antimicrobial drugs and pesticides have reduced the recurrence of such scourges as the plague. But isolated cases are still reported around the world, and outbreaks are still possible in areas where wild rodent populations are persistently infected with the plague bacillus. As the boundary areas shrink that separate suburbs and their peridomestic rodents from infected rural/wild rodent populations, the risk remains. Such regions include the western United States and parts of South America, Africa, and Asia. The last great plague epidemic occurred in the early 20th century in India and caused more than 10 million deaths. Rembrandt van Rijn's *The Rat Catcher* draws a direct line between the social ills that have always caused plague and the ingredients in modern societies that can make it happen again and again.

At mid-20th century, tuberculosis was still acknowledged as the "great white plague." The persistence of this disease in light of known prevention and treatment may be due to its greatly reduced clinical and epidemiologic importance in wealthy nations. Some believe that tuberculosis has "not really emerged so much as emerged from the ranks of the poor." When complex forces move more poor people into the United States and Western Europe, tuberculosis incidence increases. In some of the immigrants' countries of origin the annual rate of infection is up to 200 times that in the United States, and when these infected persons arrive in the United States many of them live crowded together in homeless shelters, correctional facilities, and camps for migrant workers. Amedeo Modigliani's *Self-Portrait 1919* is more than an image of the painter, who died of the disease. It is the portrait of tuberculosis.

The link between war and pestilence probably precedes the biblical Four Horsemen of the Apocalypse. Conflict and infection are closely linked. Displacement of people creates disaster conditions: large refugee populations living with compromised or nonexistent infrastructure and sanitation, contaminated water and food supplies, wound infections, and increased poverty. Conflict enhances the spread of diseases by moving people and their infections (malaria, cholera, tuberculosis) to new areas with an ample supply of susceptible people. Among US troops, infections have traditionally produced higher hospital admission rates than battle injuries and, until World War II, higher death rates. In conflicts where returning armies were quarantined to avoid spread of disease, for example, during the 1918 influenza pandemic with military personnel returning to Australia, rates of infection were substantially reduced. Pablo Picasso's iconic *Guernica* makes an antiwar statement now as it did during its first appearance in 1937.

Among the most troubling connections of conflict and disease resurfacing in the United States in the late 20th century was the intentional release of biological agents. Dissemination of anthrax spores through the postal system raised the specter of biological agent use for political or ideological reasons. Harming large groups of people in this way is an old practice that causes disease emergence. Whether involving salmonella mixed in food, anthrax distributed in the mail, or the possible use of botulinum toxins or plague bacilli, this practice is intended to terrorize populations, but in the end it contaminates the environment, food, or water with dangerous pathogens, creating disease where none need exist. Norman Rockwell's *Postman Reading Mail* could not be more to the point on the topic of unnecessary suffering. Through ironic contrast, this classic Rockwell image brings home the horror of intentional release of biological agents.

Rain comprises three parts in a nontraditional ensemble depicting one of Jaune Quick-to-See Smith's favored themes, the close bond between humanity and nature. The main part of the ensemble is a long visual field painted in somber tones and punctuated with glistening metal spoons, arranged without regularity but with internal vertical symmetry, synchronized as they are by a powerful guiding force, gravity. The colors (grays, yellows, browns, reds) smear and run, blending into each other in alternating flat patches and dark grooves that give the strands of runny paint a three-dimensional effect.

Smith's icon of suffering engages the viewer in an empathetic recall of past wrongs, from environmental degradation to cultural annihilation through, among other causes, the spread of disease. When smallpox was introduced on the North American continent, it devastated the immunologically naïve Native population. Later, the human spirit, whose survival is at the heart of 20th-century art, triumphed over the disease, eradicating it from the planet. Challenges to the bond between humanity and nature continue, emerging unpredictably and without end. Anthrax spores, fully understood and refined, were released into the US postal system, reviving the specter of intentional biologic contamination. Like scientific efforts to anticipate and curtail the threat, Smith's work confronts the pain of human and environmental catastrophe, embracing efforts to prevent it.

Bibliography

Lippard LR. *Mixed Blessings: New Art in a Multicultural America.* New York, NY: Pantheon; 1990.

National Museum of Women in the Arts. Jaune Quick-To-See Smith. Available at: http://www. nmwa.org/explore/artist-profiles/jaune-quick-see-smith. Accessed June 4, 2013.

Potter P. Biologic agents and disease emergence. Available at: http://wwwnc.cdc.gov/eid/ article/10/7/ac-1007_article.htm. Accessed June 4, 2013.

Walden J, Kaplan EH. Estimating time and size of bioterror attack. *Emerg Infect Dis.* 2004;10:1202–1205.

Walkingstick K, Marshall AE. *So Fine! Masterworks of Fine Art from the Heard Museum.* Phoenix, AZ: Heard Museum; 2001.

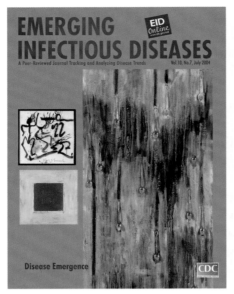

Disease Emergence; http://dx.doi.org/10.3201/eid1007.AC1007

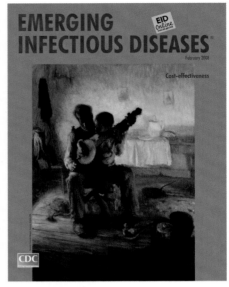

Cost-Effectiveness; http://dx.doi.org/10.3201/eid1402.AC1402

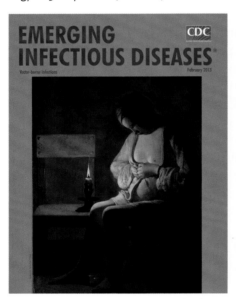

Vector-borne Infections; http://dx.doi.org/10.3201/eid1902.AC1902

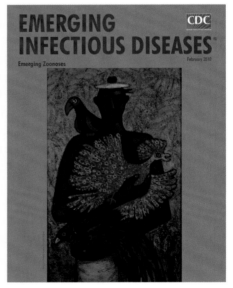

Emerging Zoonoses; http://dx.doi.org/10.3201/eid1602.AC1602

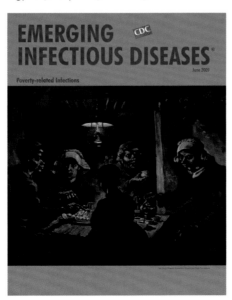

Poverty-related Infections; http://dx.doi.org/10.3201/eid1506.AC1506

EMERGING
INFECTIOUS DISEASES

EID Online
www.cdc.gov/eid

A Peer-Reviewed Journal Tracking and Analyzing Disease Trends   Vol.10, No.11, November 2004

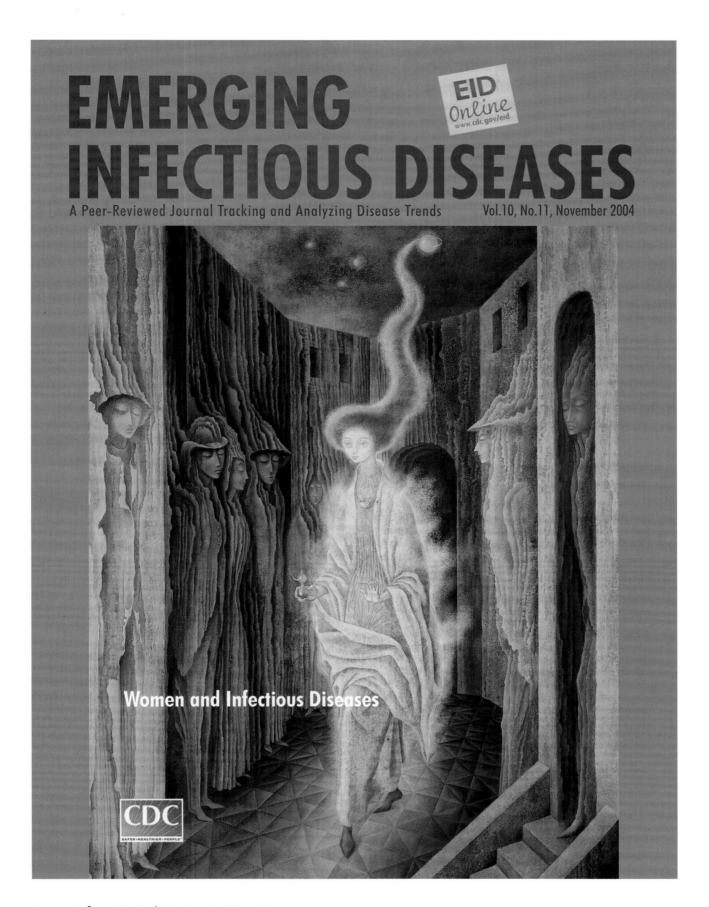

Women and Infectious Diseases

CDC

SCIENTIFIC DISCOVERY AND WOMEN'S HEALTH

"Surrealism claims totally the work of the enchantress too soon gone," said André Breton, when he heard that Remedios Varo had died, in 1963. Surrealism, which sought to express "the actual functioning of thought," was Varo's vehicle for understanding the universe, a vehicle that, like the fanciful locomotives in many of her paintings, went beyond established scientific principles. Bolstered by intuition and intellectual curiosity, the movement accessed the world of dreams, memory, and the psyche.

To this expansive world, Varo brought knowledge of engineering construction, painstaking attention to detail, a penchant for philosophical discourse, and fascination with alchemy and the occult. The result was a personal approach to surrealism, the unified vision of a fantastic world inhabited by creatures of the imagination, moving freely in and out of consciousness, proposing new solutions, offering alternative interpretations.

A native of Angles, Spain, Remedios Varo grew up in a family that nurtured academic and artistic aspirations. Her father, a hydraulics engineer, encouraged her interest in science and taught her how to draft images, a skill she used throughout her artistic career. At age 15, she enrolled in the renowned fine arts academy of San Fernando in Madrid, also attended around the same time by budding surrealist, Salvador Dalí.

At the academy, which featured such lecturers as Marie Curie, H. G. Wells, Albert Einstein, and José Ortega y Gasset, Varo became familiar with new ideas: the theories of Sigmund Freud, which broadened the boundaries of reality; and the work of André Breton, which defined surrealism as a literary and artistic movement. She was exposed to the treasures of the Prado Museum and the influences of Hieronymus Bosch, Francisco Goya, El Greco, Picasso, and Braque.

Varo's rigorous academic training formed the backbone of an artistic career marked by innovation and creativity and frequently interrupted by conflict. The Spanish Civil War forced her to flee Barcelona, where she had become part of the bohemian avant-garde, for Paris, where she apprenticed among the surrealists' inner circle and exhibited her work widely. She left Europe to escape World War II, and Mexico became the adoptive home where in the last 10 years of her life she produced the bulk of her mature work.

Mexico, with its pre-Columbian cultures, primitive art, and abundant hospitality, provided Varo broad artistic freedom and an exciting context in which to practice surrealist rebellion. Yet her first few years in exile were marked by economic hardship and emotional isolation: "We are finally installed here . . . suffering from the 2,400 meters altitude . . . dead with fatigue and having heart ailments." Away from her familiar circle, she struggled to secure what Virginia Woolf once identified as the basic requirements for an artistic career: a steady income and "a room of one's own." She painted furniture, worked for Bayer Pharmaceuticals as an illustrator, and during a brief visit to Venezuela, produced scientific drawings for that country's Ministry of Public Health.

Varo's interest in scientific discovery, reflected even in the titles of her works, extended to cosmology, evolution, astronomy, and genetics: *Phenomenon of Weightlessness,*

Cosmic Energy, Weaving of Space and Time, Creation of the Birds, Discovery of a Mutant Geologist, Exploration of the Sources of the Orinoco River, Vegetal Architecture. Her paintings showed empathetic understanding of the human condition and often contained elaborate mechanical devices and instruments of science meant to improve it.

"[A]s if she paints with her gaze rather than her hands, Remedios clears the canvas and over its transparent surface she gathers simple truths," said Mexican poet Octavio Paz in his poem "Apparitions and Disappearances." Her protagonists, who bear her heart-shaped face, almond eyes, long sharp nose, and abundant hair, move in a metaphysical world. As they straddle the line between real and unreal, they seem aware of their demands on the viewer's imagination. Witty and engaging, they levitate in narrative scenes filled with fantastic plant and animal life. Some cats are so wild they are made of ferns, some women so domesticated they have chair arms and chair legs.

The Call is inhabited by apparitions and has the eerie stillness and depthless unreality of a dream. A flaming female figure charged by a celestial body emanates energy and lights up the scene; around her neck, a single ornament, a chemist's mortar; in her hand, a laboratory flask, a retort. The lurid presence casts a glow on the dim walls of a hallway. From these walls, like a hallucinogenic distortion, a mournful array of human forms bulge forward, feet anchored to the floor, eyes downcast, bodies lost in outlandish folds: female phantoms, pillars and structural support, trapped in a paralyzing nightmare.

Mysterious and provocative, the architectural stage is cluttered with conflicting clues. The walls are tall; the windows small and out of reach; the sky inflamed; the morbid folds props of oppression. Yet the floor is elaborately tiled, the doorways arched, the steps well tended. The stage is firmly cast; oppression is institutionalized.

Varo's enigmatic *Call*, part dream part symbolic reality, seems at once a calling and a call to action. The flaming figure wears the signs and halo of science. Bathed in the light of knowledge, she steps forward boldly to dispel the darkness. In the painter's surreal universe as well as ours, the female phantoms on the wall stand for poverty, confinement, disease. Overlooked by societies, biomedical research, and health care systems; battered by AIDS, malaria, and other infections; victimized by globalization; and stigmatized by the very diseases that confine and kill them, women slumber in the shadows. The flaming figure's flask contains the science. Her call is a wake-up call.

Bibliography

Bellamy C. Globalization and infectious diseases in women. *Emerg Infect Dis.* 2004;10: 2022–2024.

Kaplan JA. *Remedios Varo: Unexpected Journeys.* New York, NY: Abbeville Press; 1988.

Lozano L-M. *The Magic of Remedios Varo.* Baltimore, MD: Schmitz Press; 2000.

Wach K. *Salvador Dalí: Masterpieces from the Collection of the Salvador Dalí Museum.* New York, NY: Harry N. Abrams, Inc.; 1996.

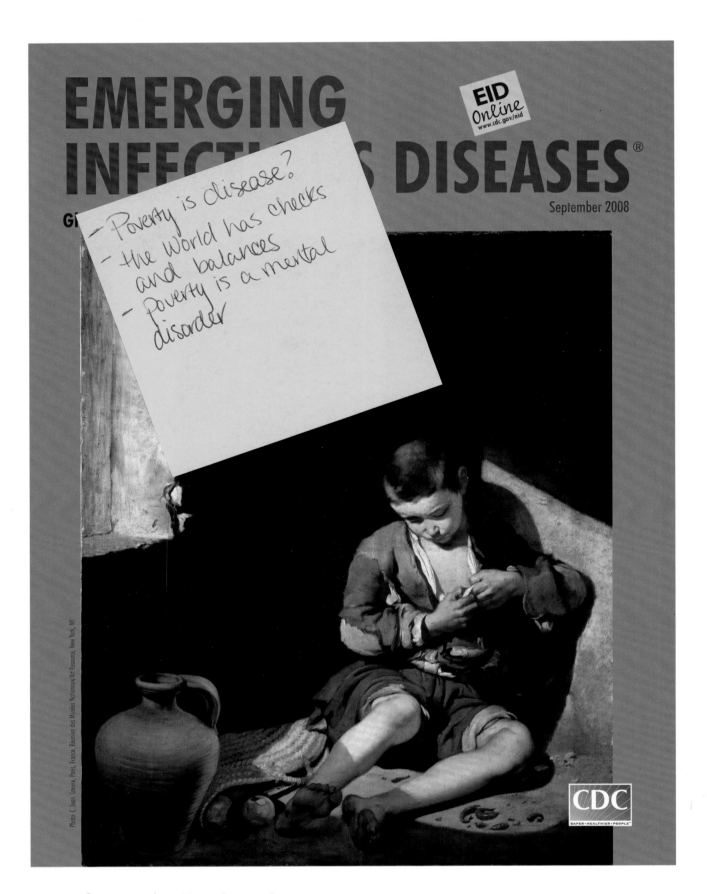

HOW COMES IT, ROCINANTE, YOU'RE SO LEAN? I'M UNDERFED, WITH OVERWORK I'M WORN[1]

"There are only two families in the world, the Haves and the Haven'ts," wrote Miguel de Cervantes (1547–1616) at a time he viewed as "no golden age" in his native Spain. A brilliant satirist, Cervantes ridiculed the socially divisive mores of a gilded imaginary past held onto for too long and seeming all the more incongruous amidst the poverty and oppression of his own life.

Spain in the 17th century, its empire collapsed and population ravaged by three plague epidemics, was embroiled in conflict abroad and royal mismanagement at home. Its misadventures, chronicled in the plays of Lope de Vega and Calderón, also fueled the genius of Diego Velázquez, Francisco de Zurbarán, Jusepe de Ribera, and Bartolomé Esteban Murillo. They, too, advanced the cultural front by constructing from the rabble a Spanish school of painting for the ages.

Spanish baroque, as the school came to be known, expanded on similar art movements in the Netherlands and elsewhere in Europe. Immortalizing royals and street peddlers alike, it left a vivid record of the times. Among the greats of this period, Murillo, a native of Seville known as much for his good character as his artistic talent, painted the indigent and populated lofty religious scenes with ordinary human faces.

Orphaned in childhood, Murillo was raised by relatives. He apprenticed under Juan del Castillo, a leading painter of the 1630s and 1640s who, along with Alonso Cano, influenced his early work. He left this apprenticeship to go into business for himself, creating popular pictures for quick sale. As a street artist, he saw the poorest in the city, so his early paintings were sympathetic portraits of the ragged boys and flower girls of Seville. His break came with a commission to paint 11 works for a local Franciscan monastery. These paintings brought him fame, and soon he was affluent enough to marry well.

He traveled to Madrid, where he likely became familiar with the work of Velázquez, fellow Sevillian and painter to the king, and the work of Rubens, Titian, Veronese, and Tintoretto in the royal galleries. He returned to his hometown to found the Seville Academy of Art, paint major works, and enjoy great popularity, even outside Spain. His mature paintings were mostly religious. Some were genre scenes with children, a novel theme. A few were fine portraits. All attained such lightness and refinement they were labeled "vaporous."

Even now, a "Murillo" stands for a good painting in Spain. The artist made an impression, although his fortunes faltered over time. His works sold so well that the king limited their export. But they were copied too often. Poor imitations in a flooded market damaged his reputation, especially since he never signed or dated his paintings.

One legend has it that Murillo died poor; another, that he gave his wealth to charitable causes. His last work, *The Espousal of St. Catherine*, commissioned for a Capuchin monastery in Cadiz, was not completed. The painter fell from the scaffold

---

1 Cervantes, *Don Quixote*.

and was severely injured. He was taken back to Seville, where his death was attributed to these injuries. *The Young Beggar* exemplifies Murillo's technique. It showcases the masterful brushwork, use of chiaroscuro, meticulous attention to naturalism, and gentleness toward his subjects that attracted the attention of later artists, among them 18th- and 19th-century's Sir Joshua Reynolds, John Constable, and Édouard Manet.

"Masterless children," a common sight in Seville, were pitied and loathed by local society, which gave them alms with one hand and dismissed them with the other. Survival and socialization on the street suited them for servile tasks, which inevitably led to adult criminal opportunities, gambling, and prostitution. In 1593, the city was "full of small boys who wander about lost and begging and dying of hunger and sleep in doorways and on stone benches by the walls, poorly dressed, almost nude, and exposed to many dangers . . . and others have died of freezing by dawn."

An unpublished parish-by-parish survey of the "honorable poor" of Seville in 1667 found that untended children aggregated in courtyards and abandoned buildings. Exposed to weather and pests, unwashed and malnourished, they were susceptible to infectious diseases, from ringworm to bubonic plague. When, against all odds, it snowed twice in 1624 and 1626, they were decimated. One study in the parish of San Bernardo showed that 27% of burials in 1617 to 1653 were of children.

Seville's population declined in the 17th century. A 1679 silk merchants' quarter survey showed that 40% of the buildings were vacant. Two serious plague epidemics and extensive emigration to the New World reduced the number of children. Charity, documented in literary works and prominent in the paintings of Murillo, was thought as noble and pious, but the ugliness of want (festered wounds, parasites, filth) so vivid in these paintings exposed the dark side. The poor had to register for licensed begging to be protected from impostors that would take "alms from the truly poor who cannot work." City authorities used charitable funds to create "hospitals" for vagrants to be put away from the public eye.

A slant of light reminiscent of Caravaggio (1571–1610) illuminates Murillo's *Young Beggar*, allowing a glimpse of his life. Weary and resigned, the boy leans against the wall, his belongings strewn along with the remnants of a meal, scraps of fish and rotting fruit. He is delousing himself. The mild demeanor of the child is punctuated by the furrowed brow and soiled feet. Like Rocinante, he is underfed, overworked, and riddled with pests.

"The Haves and the Haven'ts" are still at it. The Haves contributing to charity, the Haven'ts flooding the streets, some 100 million of them around the globe: migrant workers in People's Republic of China and elsewhere, homeless in Los Angeles, Bristol, or Marseille. Authorities still sort the truly and deserving poor from impostors, while the ugliness of want (lice, tuberculosis, flu, HIV/AIDS, hepatitis, diphtheria) is not shrinking from public view.

The pathos in Murillo's *Young Beggar* lies in the child's complete abandon and his charm, unblemished by the circumstances. Well addressed in literature and art, the plight of the poor, its abatement and elimination, is a main concern of public health. Armed with time-honored public health practice: health education, prescription and device distribution, tuberculosis screening and treatment, improved hygiene, ivermectin use against scabies and body louse infestation, and systematic immunization, the public health worker can now join other dreamers championed by Cervantes in declaring, "'My armour is my only wear, / My only rest the fray'."

Bibliography

Badiaga S, Raoult D, Brouqui P. Preventing and controlling emerging and reemerging transmissible diseases in the homeless. *Emerg Infect Dis.* 2008;14:1353–1359.

Cervantes M. *Don Quixote.* Ormsby J, trans. Norwalk, CT: The Heritage Press; 1950.

Jia Z-W, Jia X-W, Liu X-L, et al. Spatial analysis of tuberculosis cases in migrants and permanent residents, Beijing, 2000–2006. *Emerg Infect Dis.* 2008;14:1413–1420.

Kubler K, Soria M. *Art and Architecture in Spain and Portugal and Their American Dominions, 1500 to 1800.* Baltimore, MD: Penguin Books; 1959.

Lassaigne J. *Spanish Painting from Velázquez to Picasso.* Gilbert S, trans. Geneva, Switzerland: Skira; 1952.

Perry ME. Crime and society in early modern Seville "Children of the Streets." Available at: http://libro.uca.edu/perry/csms9.pdf. Accessed July 14, 2008.

Perry ME. Crime and society in early modern Seville "Beggars and Benefactors." Available at: http://libro.uca.edu/perry/csms8.htm. Accessed July 14, 2008.

Vol 13, No 6, June 2007

DEPARTMENT OF
HEALTH & HUMAN SERVICES
Public Health Service
Centers for Disease Control and Prevention (CDC)
Atlanta, GA 30333

EMERGING INFECTIOUS DISEASES®

EID Online
www.cdc.gov/eid

June 2007

Emerging Microbial Hazards

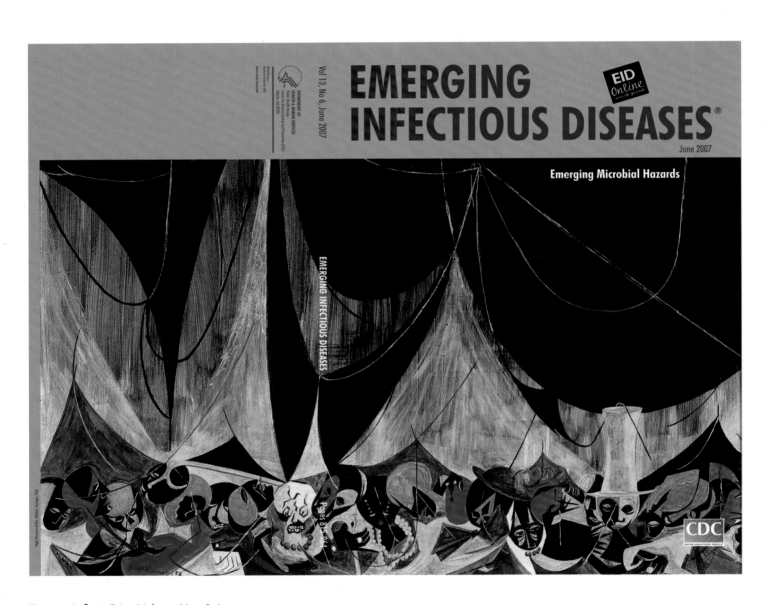

EMERGING INFECTIOUS DISEASES

Pages 815–964

CDC
SAFER · HEALTHIER · PEOPLE™

WHAT DID I DO TO BE SO BLACK AND BLUE?[2]

"Our homes were very decorative, full of . . . pattern . . . color. . . . The people used this as a means of brightening their life," said Jacob Lawrence, attributing his love of vibrant color design to his youth in Harlem. When asked whether anyone in his family was artistically inclined, he would say no: "It's only in retrospect that I realized I was surrounded by art. You'd walk Seventh Avenue and look in the windows and you'd see all these colors in the depths of the Depression, all these colors!" "Most of my work depicts events from the many Harlems that exist throughout the United States. This is my genre. My surroundings. The people I know . . . the happiness, tragedies, and the sorrows of mankind."

Lawrence was born in Atlantic City, New Jersey. "But I know nothing about it," he always said, because his family soon moved, to Pennsylvania. He moved again in his early teens, with his mother, after his parents separated. "And we came to New York and of course this was a completely new visual experience." Lawrence showed artistic talent at an early age. "I liked design. . . . I used to do things like rugs by seeing the pattern . . . in very bright primary and secondary colors . . . and papier-mâché masks . . . not for play or anything . . . I just liked to make them. . . . My first exposure to art which I didn't realize was even art at the time was at an after-school settlement house. . . . The Utopia Children's Settlement House."

"I never saw an art gallery until I was about eighteen years of age. . . . And going to the settlement house I was exposed to arts and crafts; soap carving, leather work, woodwork and painting." In the early 1930s, Depression relief programs sprang up all over the United States. Lawrence met Augusta Savage, already a well-known sculptor, at a center across the street from where he lived. He met writers Alain Locke, Richard Wright, and Ralph Ellison and worked with many prominent artists of the day, Norman Lewis, Charles Alston, Romare Bearden, Henry Bannarn.

Encouraged by Augusta Savage, he participated in the Works Progress Administration's Federal Arts Project, a program founded in 1935 to create jobs in the arts, "[I]t was like a very informal schooling. You were able to ask questions of people who had more experience . . . about technical things in painting." For inspiration, he visited the 135th Street Branch of the New York Public Library and walked 60 blocks to the Metropolitan Museum of Art.

Lack of academic training did not thwart Lawrence's artistic development. Rather, his individual style, borne of his personal view of the world and nourished by the community around him, flourished early and well. His flat patterns and colors and bold narrative scenes showed the influence of Mexican painters José Clemente Orozco, David Alfaro Siqueiros, and Diego Rivera, and of Polish artist Käthe Kollwitz, all of whom espoused a social realist philosophy.

At age 21, Lawrence attracted attention with his series of 41 paintings on Toussaint Louverture (c. 1743–1803), a hero of the Haitian Revolution. He read voraciously and researched his topics thoroughly. He painted a story over a series of panels planned and executed as a cluster. Each scene was outlined in pencil, each

---

2 Louis Armstrong. Lyrics, Andy Razaf. Music, "Fats" Waller and Harry Brooks.

color applied to all panels simultaneously to ensure consistent tonal quality across the series.

"The Human subject is the most important thing. My work is abstract in the sense of having been designed and composed, but it is not abstract in the sense of not having human content . . . I want to communicate. I want the idea to strike right away." Lawrence freed his figures of detail, exacting the essence, which he punctuated with saturated color recalling Henri Matisse, and he repeated patterns and breaks, creating a rhythmic quality reminiscent of jazz syncopations. In gouache and tempera, he re-created the "hard, bright, and brittle" feel of Harlem during the Great Depression.

The work that brought Lawrence national recognition was *The Migration of the Negro*, a series of 60 panels recounting the mass movement of African Americans from the rural South to northern urban centers. The series was featured in *Fortune* magazine in 1941. He continued to paint for decades, at times doubting the strength of his style within modernism and questioning the influence of popularity on his work. He taught at the Pratt Institute, the New School for Social Research in New York, the Skowhegan School of Painting and Sculpture in Maine, and the University of Washington in Seattle. When he died at 82, Lawrence the chronicler of major cultural events of the 19th and 20th centuries had created an American aesthetic, and his expressive style, crafted in Harlem workshops, had made a lasting impression.

In *Marionettes*, Lawrence revisited a topic addressed in *The Dancing Doll* (1947), an earlier work he had described as "mostly autobiographical." *Marionettes*, controlled with strings by a puppeteer from above, predate live theater. They were found in the tombs of ancient Egypt and the works of Archimedes and Plato.

Their inherent inability to stand alone makes marionettes an irresistible artistic and literary metaphor. In *Invisible Man* (1947), his epic of self-discovery, Ralph Ellison describes his encounter with a marionette: "I'd seen nothing like it before. A grinning doll of orange-and-black tissue paper with thin flat cardboard disks forming its head and feet and which some mysterious mechanism was causing to move up and down in a loose-jointed, shoulder-shaking, infuriatingly sensuous motion, a dance that was completely detached from the black, mask-like face."

Viewed en masse at the bottom of the painting, Lawrence's marionettes seem dwarfed under the dark backdrop and drooping tents, the inevitable strings a reminder of their attachment to a set. In what seems a makeshift theater, they await the next move. To paint the lifeless dolls, the artist was prompted by social ills, which strip people of control over their lives, causing them to withdraw because, as Ellison put it, "ain't nothing I can do but let whatever is gonna happen, happen."

As with all his work, Lawrence touched a universal nerve: human vulnerability against forces beyond one's control. "I'm so forlorn, Life's just a thorn / My heart is torn / Why was I born?" lamented Louis Armstrong (1901–1971), speaking for Lawrence and for all of us. Faced with overwhelming social injustice or with recurring insults of a more biologic nature—microbial resistance to drugs, mutating viruses, emerging prions, migrating hazards—we may at times seem little more than hapless marionettes, caught in a degrading tangle at the foot of a large set.

Bibliography

Collins AF. Jacob Lawrence: art builder. *Art Am.* 1988;2:130–135.

Ellison R. *Invisible Man.* New York, NY: Signet Books; 1952.

Lewis S. *African American Art and Artists.* Berkeley: University of California Press; 1990.

Oral history interview with Jacob Lawrence, 1968 Oct. 26. Available at: http://www.aaa.si.edu/collections/interviews/oral-history-interview-jacob-lawrence-11490. Accessed April 9, 2007.

Stella P. Modern storytellers: Romare Bearden, Jacob Lawrence, Faith Ringgold. In: *Timeline of Art History.* New York, NY: The Metropolitan Museum of Art; 2000.

Wernick R. Jacob Lawrence: art as seen through a people's history. *Smithsonian.* 1987;18:57.

EMERGING
INFECTIOUS DISEASES®

EID Online www.cdc.gov/eid

October 2007

Global Poverty

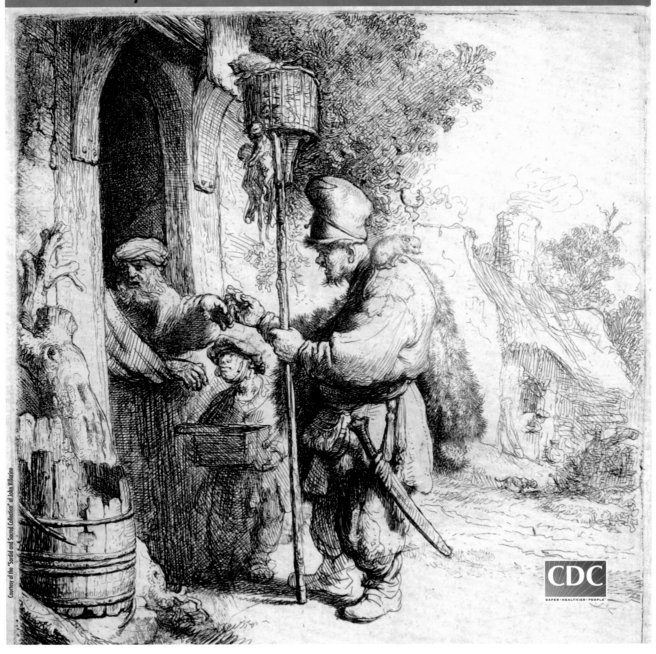

Courtesy of the "Sordid and Sacred Collection" of John Villarino

CDC
SAFER · HEALTHIER · PEOPLE™

RATS, GLOBAL POVERTY, AND PAYING THE PIPER

"I frankly consider him a great virtuoso," said Italian painter Guercino of Rembrandt van Rijn. Guercino (1591–1666) was referring to the legendary master not as painter or portraitist but as etcher because it was etchings that built Rembrandt's reputation during his lifetime. The first to fully exploit this technique, which dates back to 14th-century armor ornamentation, he left behind some 300 fine prints, a benchmark for posterity. Most were small, displayed not on walls but in albums like early photographs, rested on tables for a closer look.

Etchings are created by drawing on a resin- or wax-coated metal plate with a needle. The plate is immersed in acid, which "bites" or eats away the lines where the metal is exposed. Rembrandt viewed this technique as drawing. Attracted to its spontaneity, he practiced it throughout his career and defined it with inventiveness and flair. His genius lay in the light touch of the draftsman, not the heavy hand of the professional printmaker. Using the needle as brush or pen, he created lines that flowed across the plates, varied in texture and tone from being carved more deeply or immersed longer in the acid bath.

For even greater tonal variation, Rembrandt experimented with drypoint—drawing lines directly into the soft surface of the copper plate. These lines held more ink and formed velvety black, rich shadows. Combined etching and drypoint limited copies from a single plate, sometimes to as few as 15, from possible hundreds. His finest prints are rare and unique, even if created by a reproductive process. Unlike other 17th-century artists, who did the drawing, then turned the task over to printmakers, he did the total job himself, able to alter the drawing throughout the process and create, from the same plate, prints that were not identical. The paper used, common European white or thin absorbent, ivory-yellow or light gray Japanese, also produced remarkable variations.

On these small plates, Rembrandt etched life in his native Holland. To capture natural movement, he ran a theatrical studio, where apprentices played out gestures for each other and enacted scenes from the streets of Amsterdam and the fringes of society. Enlivened with dramatic light and shadow, these indelible scenes established his reputation as master storyteller. They described an urban culture conscious of boundaries and criteria for inclusion and exclusion; focused on work, thrift, and restraint; and overwrought with vagabonds, landlopers, beggars, tricksters, outsiders—a population both created and demonized by society and portrayed in sordid detail by period art.

Earlier painters, Hieronymus Bosch (c. 1450–1516) for one, depicted beggars as indistinguishable from demons. Peter Bruegel the Elder (c. 1525–1569) painted peasants as objects of mirth, and Adriaen van de Venne (1589–1662) capped his unsparing images of the poor with ironic humor and ridicule. Some of Rembrandt's prints show the poor in unflattering and compromising situations, but he was indebted to Jacques Callot (c. 1592–1635), whose etchings he collected. They humanized the poor and allowed them individuality and seriousness.

Rembrandt may have learned compassion from his own misfortunes. His life, which might have been one of comfort, recognition, and wealth, turned into a journey of adversity, marred by the deaths of his wife and young children, bankruptcy, and social rejection in his later years. Bitter and disillusioned, he continued to produce earthy street scenes crowded with beggars, peddlers, the underclass, whose faces were oddly reminiscent of his own portraits or those he painted in religious scenes.

In the disorderly intimacy of the streets that so fascinated Rembrandt, economic delinquency manifested itself in more than just the unwanted poor. Stray animals, a hog here and there, tame pigeons, cats, rabid dogs, roamed unchecked. And rats, most prolific, most hated and feared, for as the poet put it, "They fought the dogs and killed the cats, / and bit the babies in the cradles, / and ate the cheeses out of the vats, / And licked the cooks' own ladles."

The house rat, or black rat, arrived in Europe around more than 2,500 years ago and quickly established a commensal relationship with the locals in homes, ships, river banks, and sewers, generating brisk business for the rat poison peddlers, common street venders. The Pied Piper of Hamelin, a legend immortalized by the Brothers Grimm, recounted rat infestation so severe in that German town, in 1284, it required special intervention.

When Europe was overrun by the Black Death in 1348, Giovanni Boccaccio, who lived through it in the city of Florence, wrote in *The Decameron*, "It began with yong children, male and female, either under the armepits, or in the groine by certaine swellings, in some to the bignesse of an Apple, in others like an Egge." His description led to later speculation that the disease was bubonic plague caused by *Yersinia pestis* and spread by fleas carried by the black rat. In *A Journal of the Plague Year*, Daniel Defoe's chronicle of the great plague of London in 1665, rats were named as suspects, "All possible Endeavours were used also to destroy the Mice and Rats, especially the latter."

In *The Rat Catcher* Rembrandt's light hand scratched a telling rat's tale in a local transaction between an itinerant peddler and a homeowner. Looking on is the peddler's diminutive assistant, holding a container with rat poison or ferrets trained to hunt rats. The peddler's extended hand holds poison. The homeowner reaches from behind the half-closed double door but is repulsed. A basket on the long pole is filled with live rats. One on top is poised to jump. Others hang dead from the base. Hairy and unkempt, the peddler himself looks like a rat in his tattered furry cape and long sword. Domestic clutter frames the entrance to the cottage. Etched softly in the background is a prowling cat.

The Rat Catcher was a popular print, copied 11 times in the 17th century. The scene struck a nerve because it contained much more than a transaction on a village lane. At the threshold of this cottage, separated by the closed half door, met but remained apart, two sections of society: the rooted and the vagrant outsider. What Rembrandt managed to convey was the humanity of all, not just the squeamish owner but the vagrants too, social outcasts though they were. The assistant wears a wistful glance. The peddler, solid on his feet, has a pet perched trustingly on his shoulder.

A carrier of bubonic plague, epidemic typhus, trench fever, rat-bite fever, leptospirosis, hantavirus pulmonary syndrome, salmonella poisoning, and many other infections, the rat is still a suspect around the world, destroying as much as one-third of the global food supply each year, killing domesticated animals, damaging buildings and furnishings. Social inequity also continues, perpetuating a cycle of poverty and disease.

This cycle cannot be ignored for, as Boccaccio and Defoe reported, disease cannot be fenced out of prosperous areas. "[T]he plague bacillus never dies . . . it bides its time in bedrooms, cellars, trunks, and bookshelves," wrote Albert Camus, in *The Plague*, "and perhaps the day would come when, for the bane and the enlightening of men, it would rouse up its rats again and send them forth to die in a happy city."

Bibliography

Arbitman KJ. Rembrandt. Available at: http://www.carnegiemuseums.org/cmag/bk_issue/1997/mayjun/feat5a.htm. Accessed July 30, 2007.

Boccaccio G. *The Decameron*. Norwalk, CT: Heritage Press; 1968.

Browning R. The pied piper of Hamelin; http://www.indiana.edu/~librcsd/etest/piper/test.html; accessed August 6, 2007.

Camus A. *The Plague*. New York, NY: Vintage; 1991.

Defoe D. *A Journal of the Plague Year*. Norwalk, CT: Heritage Press; 1968.

Fleischer R, Scott SC, eds. *Rembrandt, Rubens, and the Art of Their Time*. University Park, PA: Pennsylvania State University; 1997.

Kelly T. Tricksters, vagrants and outsiders: economic delinquents in painting. Symposium session: Representation and regulation: 17th-century economics in the Dutch Republic; November 12, 2004; Amsterdam, The Netherlands.

Schwartz G. Sordid and sacred: the beggars in Rembrandt's etchings; http://www.a-r-t.xom/rembrandt/remessay.htm; accessed July 30, 2007.

Sullivan R. *Rats*. New York, NY: Bloomsbury; 2004.

Zinsser H. *Rats, Lice, and History*. New York, NY: Black Dog & Leventhal; 1996.

EMERGING

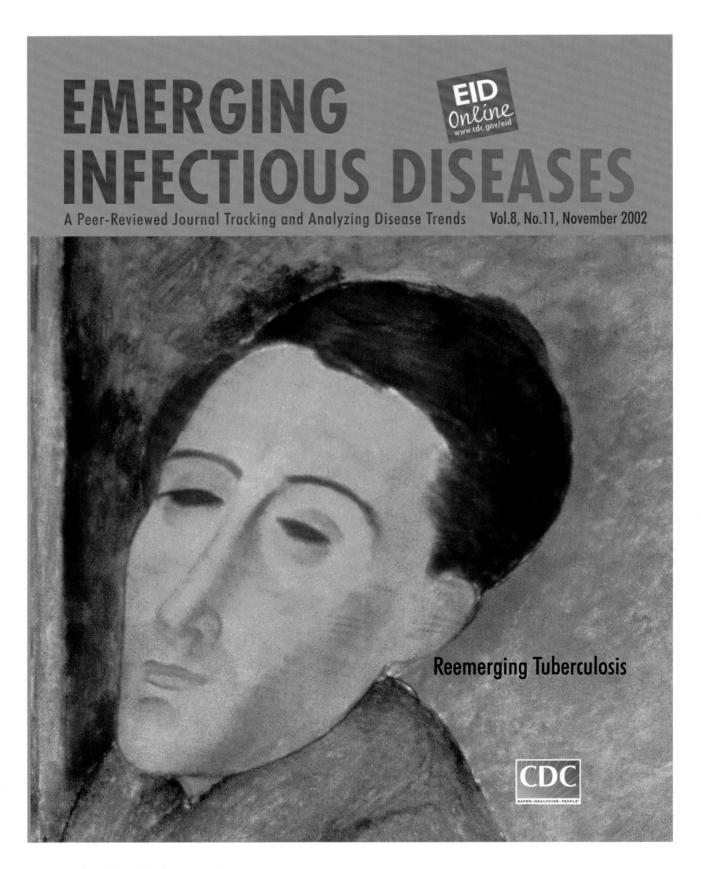

EID Online
www.cdc.gov/eid

INFECTIOUS DISEASES

A Peer-Reviewed Journal Tracking and Analyzing Disease Trends   Vol.8, No.11, November 2002

Reemerging Tuberculosis

CDC
SAFER·HEALTHIER·PEOPLE

THE FACE OF TUBERCULOSIS

Modigliani was born in Livorno, Italy, where he grew up in a Jewish ghetto. He studied art in Florence, and in 1906 he moved to Paris, where he met Pablo Picasso and other leading artists of his era. In Paris, he was influenced by fauvism, the avant-garde art movement promoting a strong, emotional, and nonrealistic use of color, and by his friend the Romanian sculptor Constantin Brancusi, known for his artistic search of pure form. Modigliani was also influenced by African carvings and masks, particularly in his early work, which was mostly sculpture.

In his brief life, which even in childhood was marked by ill health, Modigliani was able to grow as an artist and attain his own distinctive style. He is known for his graceful, simplified, and sympathetic portrayal of the human form. His paintings, mostly portraits and studies of the human figure, are characterized by fine sinuous lines and have a simple, spare, and flat appearance, which gives them an almost classical effect. The figures are elongated, the faces oval, and the shapes ethereal, reminiscent at times of Sandro Botticelli. The portraits (more than 200 from 1916 to 1919), unburdened by detail, rely on color and shape for emotional and psychological insight and emit a "curious sense of pathos."

Modigliani's fauvist contemporaries had moved away from the conventional and sentimental in art. They were not interested in the representation of observed reality or even in passion mirrored on a face. They were after "radical simplicity," the "genius of omission." Expression to them was achieved through form and spatial depth, the arrangement of line and color on a flat plane, and the empty spaces around them. In this artistic climate, Modigliani would not have been interested in tuberculosis as a subject for his art, nor would he have painted a conventional portrait of this disease that consumed his adult life and eventually killed him at age 36.

This famous *Self-Portrait*, painted in 1919, just 1 year before Modigliani's death, inspired writers who were captivated by its romanticism to speculate broadly about its meaning. Even though many of the interpretations are mostly conjecture, the length and thinness of the face, as well as its pallor and eerie calmness, may well be due to tuberculosis.

In this portrait, so reminiscent of the African masks that had fascinated him not for their intense expression but for their formal simplicity and coherence, Modigliani seems to have captured the essence of his subject, himself. He turned to his fauvist roots for the striking hues so typical of tuberculous complexion, to his friend Brancusi's sculptures for the studied serenity, and to his own emotional capacity for the depths of darkness welled in those stylized eyes. But whether he intended it or not, the master portrait painter, Modigliani, in this self-portrait of hollowed cheeks and sealed lips, painted more than his face. He painted the face of tuberculosis.

Bibliography
Chretien J. *Tuberculosis: The Illustrated History of a Disease.* Hauts-de-France; Vol. 1. Translated by Clare Pierard. Béthune, France: Hauts de France Editions, 1998.
Werner, A. *Amedeo Modigliani.* London, England: Thames and Hudson; 1967.

EMERGING
INFECTIOUS DISEASES

EID Online www.cdc.gov/eid

A Peer-Reviewed Journal Tracking and Analyzing Disease Trends   Vol.8, No.10, October 2002

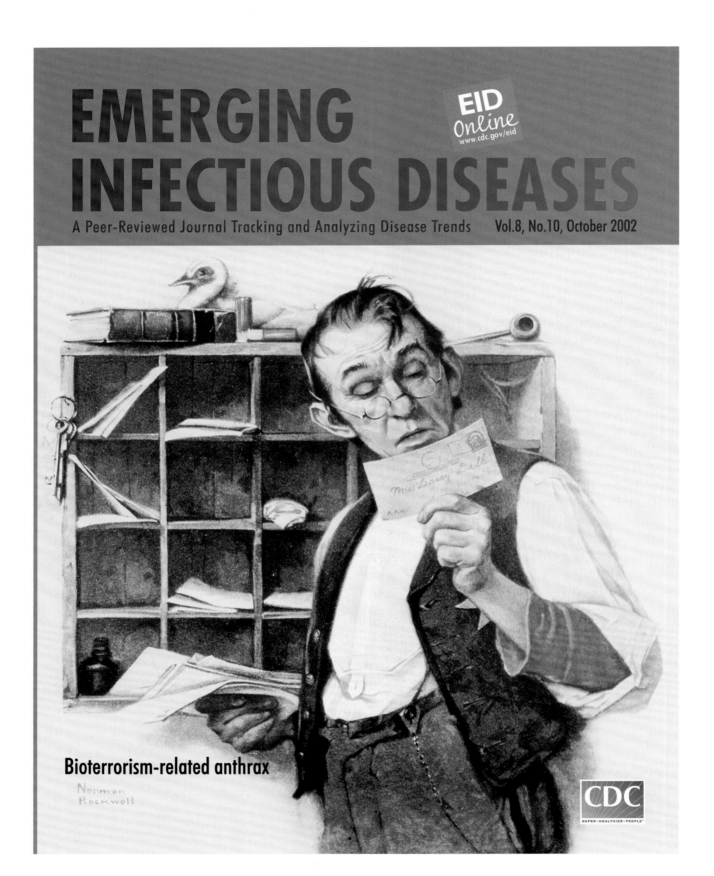

Bioterrorism-related anthrax

Norman Rockwell

CDC

Emerg. Infect. Dis., Vol. 8, No. 10, Oct. 2002

POSTAL WORK NOW AND THEN

Norman Rockwell, North America's most beloved and certainly best known illustrator, favored scenes of everyday life and reveled in his ability to tell stories. His Dickensian view of life drove him to paint the world as he would like it to be—no drunken fathers or self-centered mothers, only kindly doctors, duty-bound soldiers, and regular folks at their daily occupations. In his pictures, the sadness was wistful and the problems humorous. Rockwell, who presented himself as an illustrator rather than a fine arts painter, was also an interpreter of the classics and a recorder of history and the contemporary scene, from the Nuclear Test Ban Treaty to the civil rights movement.

The realism in Rockwell's illustrations was not photographic. Along with the artful detail, his cast of characters (teachers, students, models, homemakers) was loaded with nuances bestowed by the illustrator's genius. The characters sparkled, glowed, and communicated directly with the audience. And the message they sent was exactly the one Rockwell intended the audience to receive.

Very much in touch with his surroundings, the artist lived many of the situations that eventually became the subjects of his pictures. He painted what he knew to be the life of a child, a student, a soldier, or a workingman, whether in the Mamaroneck, New York, of his youth, or anywhere else he lived after that. As a result, his characters were universal and accessible to the average viewer.

Rockwell's brief experience with the US Postal Service, which may have colored his many depictions of postal workers of all ages, was in the eighth grade. To raise money for art school tuition, he bought the mail route to exclusive Orienta Point from another boy for $25. The wealthy residents of the Point each paid the mail carrier 25 cents to deliver the mail because the regular carrier did not deliver that far from town. Every morning at 5:30, rain or shine, Norman bicycled to the post office, loaded the mail into a leather shoulder bag, and rode 2.5 miles to the end of the Point, delivering the mail to homes on the way.

When *Postman Reading Mail* first hit the stands on the cover of the *Saturday Evening Post*, thousands of letters from postal workers protested the nosy behavior ascribed to one of their own. Rockwell fielded the protests graciously, explaining that the post office was a small operation, in a tiny town, with a few boxes of mail to sort, and the postal clerk had succumbed to boredom and human curiosity: "if you are interested in the characters that you draw, and understand them and love them, why the person who sees your picture is bound to feel the same way" (Curtis Publishing Co. comm., 2002).

If premier illustrator Norman Rockwell were alive today, he would be painting a different mail scene from the one featured on the cover of the *Saturday Evening Post* in 1922 more recently on the cover of *Emerging Infectious Diseases*. Under the current circumstances of the world, in which the routine and harmless activity of sorting and delivering the mail was deliberately contaminated with a dreaded disease, this fine recorder of history would probably forego the humor in the scene.

Bibliography
Rockwell N. *My Adventures as an Illustrator*. New York, NY: Harry Abrams; 1988.

DEPARTMENT OF
HEALTH & HUMAN SERVICES
Public Health Service
Centers for Disease Control and Prevention (CDC)
Atlanta, GA 30333

Official Business
Penalty for Private Use $300

Return Service Requested

ISSN 1080-6040

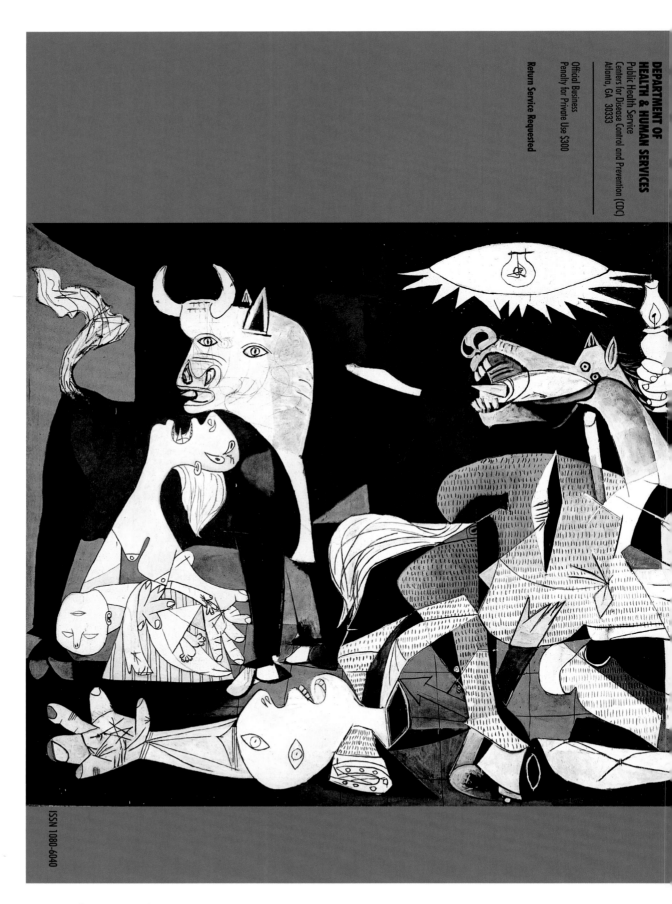

EMERGING
INFECTIOUS DISEASES

EID Online
www.cdc.gov/eid

A Peer-Reviewed Journal Tracking and Analyzing Disease Trends

Vol.9, No.6, June 2003

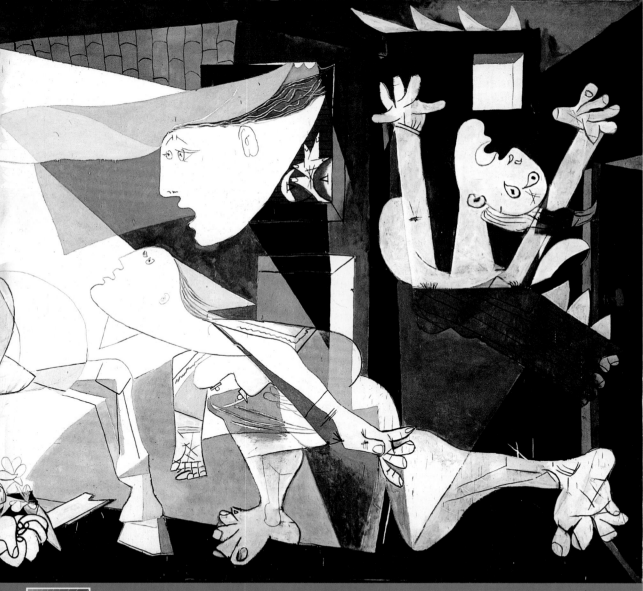

Bioterrorism-related anthrax

ART IS THE LIE THAT TELLS THE TRUTH

"It isn't up to the painter to define the symbols," said Pablo Picasso when asked to explain his celebrated mural, *Guernica*. "The public who look at the picture must interpret the symbols as they understand them." Picasso himself did not know what the work would turn out to be when he was commissioned to paint the centerpiece for the Spanish Pavilion of the 1937 World's Fair in Paris: "A painting is not thought out in advance. While it is being done, it changes as one's thoughts change. And when it's finished, it goes on changing, according to the state of mind of whoever is looking at it."

The official theme of the World's Fair was modern technology, but the inspiration for Picasso's mural came from world events—specifically the Nazi bombing and virtual obliteration of Guernica, an ancient Basque town in northern Spain. The bombardment of this nonmilitary target took little more than 3 hours, during which airplanes, plunging low from above the center of town, machine-gunned the townspeople who had taken refuge in the fields. News reports and horrific photographs of the massacre quickly reached Paris and provided the story line for perhaps the best-known painting of the 20th century. Started 6 days after the bombing and completed in 5 weeks, the monumental mural captured the agony brought on by brutality and violence.

A native of Andalusia, Spain, who lived most of his life in France, Picasso was the most innovative artist of his era and perhaps any era. His complex genius is usually tracked in a series of overlapping periods beginning in 1901. A master of classical art, he painted the poor, whose ordinary activities he imbued with melancholy and lyricism (blue period, rose period). Around 1905, influenced by Cézanne and African sculpture, he experimented with fragmented and distorted images and became one of the founders of modern abstraction, literally "the drawing away from or separating."

Destroying in order to create, Picasso dismantled traditional forms and sought the inner geometry of objects and the human figure. His *Les Demoiselles d'Avignon* (1907) marked the beginning of analytic cubism, the harsh intellectual style (also of Braque and Gris) in which decomposition of objects into geometric lines and contours is carried to an extreme. Figures and their surroundings are broken into "angular wedges or facets," shaded to appear three-dimensional. We cannot tell whether the fragments are concave or convex; some seem "chunks of modified space," others translucent bodies comprising a fantastic world of compounded voids and solids.

Traditional art confines its subject to one time and place. Cubism allows the artist to express what Albert Einstein defined in 1905 in his theory of relativity: a new sense of time, space, and energy in which moving figures become an extension of the environment from which they are indistinguishable. As art, the world, and self converge, continuity and brokenness, symmetrical progression, life and death, pain and hope can be viewed within a broader aesthetic reality. Around 1909, Picasso eliminated color, replacing it with a range of gray and brown tones to which he added new elements, paper cutouts, numbers, and letters, creating collages and other new techniques that further separated the work of art from any representation of reality. In a later form, cubism became "synthetic," more representational and flat, and included bright decorative patterns (as in *The Three Musicians*, 1921).

"Art is the lie that tells the truth," Picasso once said, articulating how an abstract painting could pack so much passion. *Guernica* does not represent the event that inspired it. Rather, in a series of allegorical images, it evokes the complexity and depth of suffering caused by the event. In a systematically crowded composition (deliberately undermining the academic rules of art), figures are crammed into the foreground: screaming mother cradling dead child, corpse with wide open eyes, arm holding lamp, fighter's arm with weapon, menacing human-faced bull, gored horse. In open darkness and surrounded by burning buildings, the figures seem united in a sublime lament, reminiscent of Mediterranean funeral rites. Their symbolism defies exact interpretation; they owe their terrific eloquence to "what they are, not what they mean." With flawless internal logic, the anatomical dislocations, fragmentations, and transformations expose the stark reality of unbearable pain.

As if conceived during a lightening strike, *Guernica* shocks in near monochrome, exemplifying the triumph of pure abstracted form. Its symbolism, punctuated by innovating techniques (e.g., inclusion of newsprint), transforms a local event to a universal icon of terror in the aftermath of violence. The figures, human and not, in primitive flight, embody the horror of living creatures under attack. With undeniable clarity, Picasso spells out in modern terms humanity's condemnation of unnecessary suffering, the agony caused not by unavoidable disasters or indecipherable diseases but by unimaginable intentional violence, such as witnessed in the deliberate release of biological agents.

Bibliography

Oppler EC, ed. *Picasso's Guernica. Norton Critical Studies in Art History.* New York: WW Norton; 1988.

Penrose R. *Picasso: His Life and Work.* London, England: Granada; 1985.

Steer G. The tragedy of Guernica: town destroyed in air attack. *The Times*, April 28, 1937. Available at: http://www.Spanish-fiestas.com/art/Picasso-guernica.htm. Accessed May 1, 2003.

Index

Page numbers in *italics* indicate illustrations.

prairie dogs, 120
prehistoric human-animal interactions, 111
primary progressive aphasia-related illness, 55–56
primates. *See* human-primate encounters
prion diseases, *138*. *See also* mad cow disease
Prison Courtyard, The (van Gogh) [Cover Sep. 2003], 150, *152*
Proust, Achille-Andrien, 128
Proust, Marcel, 128, 129
public health breakdown, poverty and, 177–178, 190
public health surveillance, xi, 56, 121
Purdy, Al, 66, 68
Pygmalion, 140

Q
Quakers, 168
quarantine, 121, 148, 150
Quest for Avuk (Machetanz) [Cover Jan. 2008], 61, 65, *67*

R
Rain (Smith) [Cover Jul. 2004], 179, *180*
Rasmussen, Knud, 66
Rat Catcher, The (Rembrandt) [Cover Oct. 2007], 178, *192*, 194
rats, 178, *192*, 193–195
Ravel, Maurice, 55
ravens, *73*, 74–75
realism, 175
reforestation, disease emergence and, 91
refugee populations, 178
regionalism, 99–100
religious sacrifice. *See* animal sacrifice
Rembrandt van Rijn
    The Rat Catcher [Cover Oct. 2007], 178, *192*, 193–195
    Scholar in His Study [Cover Mar. 2006], xiii, *xvii*
Remembrance of Things Past (Proust), 128, 129
Renaissance in the North, xiv
Renoir, Pierre-Auguste [Cover Oct. 2006], 1, *6*, 7–9
resistance. *See* antimicrobial drug resistance
respiratory infections, *98*, 100–101, *152*
Return of the Herd (Bruegel) [Cover Nov. 2007], *4*, *13*, 15
revolutions, art and music as instrument of, 52
rickettsia, fleas in transmission of, 126
Rickettsia felis, 56
Right and Left (Homer) [Cover Jan. 2006], xi–xii, *xvii*

"Rime of the Ancient Mariner, The" (Coleridge), 71
ritual sacrifice of animals. *See* animal sacrifice
Roa, Francisco [Cover Mar. 2007], 151, *174*, 175–176
Rockman, Alexis [Cover Apr. 2006], 63, *86–87*, 88–89
Rockwell, Norman [Cover Oct. 2002], 179, *198*, 199
rodents. *See* rats
Roman census, 119–120, 121, *122*
Rouault, Georges [Cover Suppl. 2001], ix, *xvii*
rowing, 95
Russian avant-garde, 150, 157
Russians knew perfectly well that the happiness of the African animals was that they had such low expectations—before the pets were introduced (Hayes), 149

S
Salmonella enterica, 162
Sands Flowers (Roa) [Cover Mar. 2007], 151, *174*, 176
SARS. *See* severe acute respiratory syndrome (SARS)
Savage, Augusta, 189
Savarin, Anthelme Brillat-, 161, 162
Schiele, Egon, *170*, 171–173
schistosomiasis, 91, 96
Schoenmaekers, M. J. H., 23
Scholar in His Study (Rembrandt) [Cover Mar. 2006], xiii, *xvii*
Schwabe, Calvin [Cover Apr. 2013], 150, 169
science, philosophic origins of, xii
scientific discovery, *181*, 182–183
scientific observation, xiv
Scream, The (Munch), 45
sea, overwhelming force of, 81–82
sea level rise, *86–87*, 88–89
Seasons, The (Bruegel), 15
Seferis, George, 164
Segal, George, 59
Self-Portrait 1919 (Modigliani) [Cover Nov. 2002], 178, *196*, 197
Self-Portrait after the Spanish Flu (Munch) [Cover Mar. 2003], 34–35, *44*, 45–46
Self-Portrait with Doctor Arrieta (Goya) [Cover May 2004], 121, *146*, 147–148
Self-Portrait with Monkey (Kahlo) [Cover Feb. 2003], 120, *131*, 132–133
Self-Portrait with Physalis (Schiele) [Cover Apr. 2013], *170*, 171–172